Synopsis of
Operative ENT Surgery

Synopsis of
Operative ENT
Surgery

Brian J. G. Bingham *FRCS(Ed)*

Consultant ENT Surgeon, Victoria Infirmary, Glasgow, UK; formerly Department of Otolaryngology, North Riding Infirmary, Middlesbrough, UK

and

Maurice R. Hawthorne *FRCS(Ed), FRCS(Eng)*

Member of the Court of Examiners, Royal College of Surgeons of England; and Consultant ENT Surgeon, North Riding Infirmary, Middlesbrough, UK

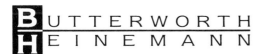

BUTTERWORTH
HEINEMANN

Butterworth-Heinemann Ltd
Linacre House, Jordan Hill, Oxford OX2 8DP

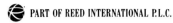 PART OF REED INTERNATIONAL P.L.C.

OXFORD   LONDON   BOSTON
MUNICH   NEW DELHI   SINGAPORE   SYDNEY
TOKYO   TORONTO   WELLINGTON

First published 1992

British Library Cataloguing in Publication Data

Bingham, Brian J. G.
  Synopsis of Operative ENT Surgery
  I. Title   II. Hawthorne, Maurice R.
  617.5

ISBN 0 7506 1359 9

Typeset by Bath Typesetting Ltd., Bath
Printed in Great Britain at the University Press, Cambridge

Contents

Preface

There is little doubt that surgery is an art and each exponent has personal techniques that achieve the best results for that individual. Consequently there are many subtleties which can only be learned by seeing the art in practice. Therefore we urge all the readers of this little book to seize every opportunity to watch their colleagues and elders at work.

Many sources have been consulted for material that has been compiled into this text. We would like to acknowledge the help that we have obtained from those texts edited by Mr John Ballantyne, Mr Andrew Morrison, Sir Donald Harrison and written by Dr J. F. Birrel, revised by Dr D. L. Cowan and Dr A. I. G. Kerr. There are many others too numerous to mention to whom we are indebted, whose work has been a source for the techniques described and illustrated in this work. We hope this book will inspire those trainees who read it to explore the greater and more comprehensive works that this synopsis is based on.

We owe a tremendous debt of thanks to the artists and authors who have agreed to have their work reproduced in the synoptic style of this book. The authors are indebted to Mr Stuart Mills, the artist who drew many of the illustrations in the text. He has tried with great difficulty to maintain a style throughout the book despite many of the illustrations having been reproduced from other texts. Out thanks also go to Peter Clarke for his photographic skills.

We would like to acknowledge our own trainers from the ENT departments of the Universities of Bristol, Manchester, Dundee, Toronto and Zurich, Selly Oak Hospital (Birmingham), Royal United Hospital (Bath), Royal Free Hospital (London) and the National Hospital for Nervous Diseases (London). It is impossible to list all those who have contributed to our training but there are several that require special mention. Firstly, Mr John Ballantyne CBE and Mr John Groves who encouraged Maurice Hawthorne to write his first book in 1983 as a registrar recently culminating in co-authorship with Roger Gray of the fifth edition of *A Synopsis of Otolaryngology*. Secondly, Professor Michael Hawke and Professor Ugo Fisch for their friendship and hospitality when the authors worked in their departments. Finally Mr Kenneth Harrison, formerly of the Manchester Royal Infirmary, who has recently died, will be remembered. He was known as 'father' by many who trained under him including Maurice Hawthorne, his last houseman.

Finally it is worth remembering that the best method of obtaining perfect wound healing is not to operate!

BJGB
MRH

Acknowledgements

The sources of many of the illustrations in this book are as follows.

J. R. Salaman and M. E. Foster, *Operative General Surgery*, Wright, London, 1988.
J. F. Birrell, *Paediatric Otolaryngology* (2nd edn), Wright, London, 1986.
J. C. Ballantyne and D. F. N. Harrison (Eds), *Rob and Smith's Operative Surgery: Nose and Throat* (4th edn) Butterworths, London, 1986.
J. C. Ballantyne and A. Morrison (Eds), *Rob and Smith's Operative Surgery: Ear* (4th edn), Butterworths, London, 1986.

Key to abbreviations of the above titles used in this book:
Operative General Surgery: OGS.
Paediatric Otolaryngology: PO.
Rob and Smith, Nose and Throat: RSN.
Rob and Smith, Ear: RSE.

Chapter 1

Preparing for surgery

PATIENT SELECTION

Most operations performed in ENT surgery are not life-saving but are aimed at improving the quality of the patient's existence. Consequently, the risks of the operation, the pain and suffering involved, and the social disruption caused by an operation have to be balanced against the possible benefits that the patient may obtain. Before agreeing to operate the surgeon should consider the following factors:

1. Physical and mental fitness of the patient.
2. Social disruption to the patient and his or her family. A long period of absence from work may jeopardize a patient's job.
3. The pain and distress caused by the operation, which may be worse than the condition.
4. The likely success rate of the operation.
5. Potential risks of damaging the patient.
6. The effectiveness of less hazardous forms of treatment.
7. The natural history of the disorder and the likelihood that a natural recovery could take place within a reasonable period of time.

Once the surgeon is convinced that an offer of surgery is merited it should be discussed with the patient. This usually takes place in the out-patient clinic. It is vitally important that the patient's expectations are ascertained since what the patient wants may be impossible to deliver. The factors listed above should be discussed with the patient. The patient should then be allowed to decide that an operation is in his or her best interest. It is important that the risks of surgery are discussed with the patient. However, these risks should not be presented in such a way that forces the patient to refuse surgery and consequently to end up in a markedly worse state of health.

PATIENT ADMISSION AND EXAMINATION

The routine admission

The patient must be given adequate notice of the admission date so that his or her personal life can be organized. A patient who is worried about social or business cares is not in an optimal state for surgery. Furthermore, there should be no doubt as to the nature of prescribed medication prior to admission. If necessary, other specialists and the patient's family doctor may have to be involved prior to the patient's admission to ensure that the patient is in the best physical and mental state for the operation.

The ward doctor should:

1. Take a history and examine the patient.
2. Liaise with the anaesthetist concerning:
   - Fitness for anaesthesia.
   - Preparation for theatre, including pre-medication.
   - Planned post-operative care.
3. Establish that the patient still requires surgery. If there are doubts then the case should be discussed with the patient's surgeon.
4. Ensure that all the results of any pre-operative investigations are available in the operating room, including blood tests, audiograms and radiographs.
5. Establish if any cross-matched blood will be required for the operation and ensure that it is available.
6. Establish and forewarn operating team members if there are any special requirements for the surgery such as:
   - Frozen section analysis.
   - Per-operative radiography.
   - Special surgical tools or implants.
   - Electrophysiological monitoring.
7. If the duty of obtaining written consent has been delegated to the ward doctor then this person must understand the proposed procedure, its risks and the likely outcome. If there are any doubts then these should be discussed with the surgeon.
8. Accurate and neat written records should be kept of all the above factors.
9. After liaison with the surgeon the ward doctor should prepare a written operating list and ensure its delivery to all departments and individuals involved.

The anaesthetist should:

1. Confirm that the patient is fit for the surgery proposed.
2. Ensure that consent has been obtained.
3. Ensure that the ward doctor has obtained all the appropriate investigations and results.
4. Plan the pre- and post-operative care, including intensive care if required.
5. Confirm that all necessary anaesthetic equipment is available and in good working order.

The surgeon should:

1. Ensure that the ward doctor has performed the duties listed above.
2. Ensure that the anaesthetist is content to proceed with the surgery.
3. Ensure that all necessary investigation results, equipment, implants and facilities are available.

4. Obtain written consent from the patient.
5. Ensure that adequate arrangements have been or can be made for post-operative care in hospital and afterwards when the patient is discharged.

The emergency admission

In the emergency situation the basic procedures for preparing a patient for surgery, as outlined under routine admission procedure, are still required. However, the time allowed for these preparations is usually reduced because of the nature of the illness. The surgeon must decide the optimal time for surgical intervention.

On the one hand, immediate intervention may be required, such as in the case of an obstructed airway. In this situation there may be no time to obtain any consent or even obtain the help of an anaesthetist. It may be only possible to obtain a brief history and to do sufficient examination to diagnose the airway obstruction before treatment is instituted to prevent death.

On the other hand, say concerning a child with a foreign body in the ear, there is the time necessary to carry out all the preparations, just as if the admission had been routine.

It is vitally important that the patient's fitness for anaesthesia is assessed. Haemorrhage should be arrested and the airway secured. Hypovolaemic shock should be identified and corrected. Biochemical abnormalities should be sought and rectified.

THE CHILD IN HOSPITAL

The special needs of children in hosptial should be recognized. These include:

1. Parental support

Where possible, accommodation should be provided for the parent to stay with the child. There should be only the minimum of restrictions on parental access to the child.

2. Education

The child requiring long-term (in excess of 2 weeks) hospital stay should be provided with school work, ideally under the guidance of a qualified teacher. Children under school age benefit from the stimulation provided by a nursery nurse.

3. Nursing

Experienced children's nurses should provide nursing care. Such people have the skill to reassure the frightened child as well as the ability to recognize the psychological and medical problems that can arise in children.

4.   *Children's ward*

Children should not be managed on a ward with adults. They need the special play facilities of a paediatric ward, and besides, sick adults are often poorly tolerant of children. Children in hospital with ENT problems are usually fit and fairly healthy. Consequently they should be nursed on an ENT paediatric ward. It can be disturbing for a child in hospital for tonsillectomy to have to share a ward with children who are dying.

From time to time deprived or abused children may fall into the care of the ENT surgeon. Children who are in the care of the local authority should be identified in order that operative consent can be given by the legal guardian. Where possible, the natural parents of such children should be kept informed. Occasionally the ward doctor or surgeon may be suspicious that a child is being physically abused or neglected. In this situation it is mandatory that a specialist experienced in these matters is consulted, ideally before the matter is mentioned to the parents. This usually means contacting a paediatrician. If such help is not immediately available it may be necessary to contact the local Social Services Department or the police. Careful notes and drawings of suspected non-accidental injuries should be made. Photographs may also be helpful. Black eyes, fractured noses and traumatic ear drum perforations are usually caused by innocent accidents and rarely deliberately. However, bruising, burns or scalds in unusual parts of the body should alert the careful doctor. A radiographic skeletal survey may be helpful.

MEDICAL RECORDS

These consist of:

1.   Written medical and nursing staff notes.
2.   Drug and fluid prescription charts.
3.   Results of investigations:
     - Blood tests.
     - Radiology reports.
     - ECG reports.
     - Neurophysiological test reports.
     - Audiological tests.
     - Special tests and reports, e.g. sweat tests.
4.   Operation records and consent forms.
5.   Anaesthetic records.
6.   Letters.
7.   Radiographs.
8.   Recordings of physiological tests.

Medical records fall into two basic categories: statements of fact and observation and statements of opinion. They should be clearly legible and every entry should be signed and dated. These records should be kept meticulously. The following information should be recorded:

1.   Demographic information.
2.   Opinion of the referring doctor.
3.   History and examination findings.

4. Conclusions drawn and the action taken:
   - Treatment instigated.
   - Investigations ordered.
5. Investigation results and action taken:
   - Treatment instigated.
6. Explanation of the diagnosis and treatment.
7. Explanation of the risks and side-effects of treatment.
8. Explanation of the risks of non-treatment.
9. Consent of the patient to advised action.
10. Details of the actual treatment and progress, including surgery.
11. Copies of letters supplying information to all parties involved, especially the family doctor.

These records should ideally be kept for as long as the patient is alive lest the information they contain is required to help manage any future illness. For legal reasons it may be necessary to keep the medical records for as long as 25 years (in the case of children) after the patient was last reviewed. However, the storage of vast numbers of records can pose a problem to many hospitals. Microfilming the notes can help in this matter. The cost benefit of reclaiming the silver from old radiographs usually means that radiographs are rarely kept longer than 6 years. Before these records are destroyed the surgeon must be satisfied that there is no risk of them being required.

In the event of a legal claim being lodged against the hospital authority or any individual involved in the care of the patient the records will be consulted. Consequently they are the main defence that the surgeon has against unjust claims of negligence. On the other hand, when a patient has been damaged as a result of a negligent act the records should help to ensure a speedy settlement and the patient's receipt of appropriate compensation.

CONSENT

Consent does not have to be written. The action of the patient can imply consent. For example, if the doctor approaches a patient with a dental syringe full of anaesthetic, tells the patient that he or she wishes to administer an anaesthetic to the gum and the patient opens his or her mouth, this action by the patient implies consent. Without consent the doctor is committing an assault. It is wise to have a written record should there be any doubt.

Consent should be informed. In England, medical negligence is handled under the system of tort. One of the arguments used by claimants is that they would not have agreed to an operation had they been fully informed of the risks. Consequently the climate of legal opinion changes as to the meaning of informed consent as the result of court actions. The wise doctor should therefore be aware of what risks are mentioned to patients by a substantial body of fellow practitioners. Should the surgeon choose to deviate from this course there must be good reason. For example, a surgeon may normally warn a patient of the risks of facial nerve paralysis in mastoid surgery, but may choose not to in a patient with an extensive cholesteatoma who might refuse surgery should they know of this risk.

There are no commonly accepted written guidelines of what risks patients should have explained. The surgeon therefore has to seek information from colleagues and from published information produced by professional insurers.

Provided the patient agrees, it is useful to involve relatives in the discussions concerning treatment. A relative who is satisfied with the patient's management is unlikely to cause trouble should the patient not have the expected outcome.

At the time of obtaining consent the operation should be discussed under the following headings:

1. Necessity of the surgery.
2. Timing of the surgery.
3. Pre- and post-operative course.
4. The proposed operation.
5. Effects on lifestyle and work.
6. Complications.

COMPLICATIONS

It is not the aim of this book to give an exhaustive list of all the complications that can arise with each operation. However, we have tried to give a list of all the common and serious risks that may arise specific to an operation.

General complications

1.   Anaesthetic

- Related to the general physical state of the patient, e.g. post-operative pulmonary problems.
- Idiosyncratic reaction to drugs.
- Misuse of drugs and anaesthetic gases. Inappropriate dosage.
- Faulty equipment, e.g. faulty valves.
- Poor technique, especially related to intubation, e.g.
  - palatal bruising
  - retropharyngeal haematoma
  - laryngeal trauma
  - oesophageal intubation
  - dental damage
- Throat packs left in place.

It is important that the general health of the patient is considered when planning surgery. The surgeon must work closely with the anaesthetist. The anaesthetist should be aware of the nature of the surgery planned and the surgeon's requirements. This is vitally important in surgery of the airway.

The surgeon must always ask permission of the anaesthetist to administer any drug, e.g. cocaine to the nose or local anaesthetic with adrenalin infiltration.

2.   Wrong operation

- Wrong patient, wrong side, wrong operation. Sadly this continues to be a problem. Every theatre should have formal procedure to prevent this problem which involves the ward, theatre and anaesthetic staff. The surgeon should always check the patient, the written consent form and the side the operation is to be performed on. It is useful to mark with a skin pen the side of the operation while the patient is awake on the ward.

3. *Failure of equipment*

   • The surgeon or his or her 'scrub' nurse should ensure that all the required instruments, implants and equipment are available and serviceable.
   • Rarely an instrument may fail or break during an operation. Every effort should be made to retrieve any fragments that may have fallen into the patient. Radiographs may help. If essential equipment fails (e.g. lighting) and a substitute cannot be found then it may be necessary to abandon the operation.
   • It is crucial that functioning suction and lighting are available before commencing any surgery, not only in the theatre but also in the recovery room.

4. *Swabs and instruments left inside the patient*

   • Prior to starting surgery and throughout the operation all swabs should be counted and recorded. This is particularly important in ear surgery, where small woolly balls may be used. These balls do not contain radio-opaque material (unlike conventional swabs) and are therefore not detectable on a plain radiograph. It is useful for swabs that are placed in 'hidden' places to have 'tails' stitched to them which can be led out onto the surface, e.g. post-nasal space swabs and neurosurgical patties.

   • A pre- and post-operative instrument count should be performed. This must include all blades and needles. The state of repair of the instruments should be assessed. A disposable tooth guard can come off a gag or an olive end from a Yankauer sucker.

5. *Theatre contamination and patient infection*

   • Failure of the ventilation system or its contamination may lead to post-operative infection.
   • Contamination of the water supply.
   • The theatre may be contaminated by an infected patient. To prevent cross-infection such patients must be identified and the theatres cleaned adequately after their surgery.
   • The theatre and medical staff should be free of infectious disease.
   • Access to theatre should be limited to essential personnel.

6. *Blood transfusion*

   • Haemolytic reactions due to incompatibility.
   • Transmission of disease, e.g. hepatitis, AIDS.

- Allergic reactions.
- Idiopathic respiratory disease syndrome. This is associated with large transfusions of non-filtered blood.
- Chilling of the patient. This occurs when large volumes of blood are infused quickly without being warmed.
- Citrate toxicity. This occurs in rapid transfusions. The treatment is to give calcium gluconate.
- Circulatory overload.
- Pyrexia due to infused pyrogens.
- Transfusion of infected blood may lead to septicaemia.

7. *Transplants and implants*

- Increased risk of infection.
- Transmission of disease. Dura carries the risk of transmitting Creutzfeld Jacob disease.
- Foreign body reaction
- Allergic reaction.
- Extrusion.
- Rejection.
- Graft versus host disease.

8. *Dressings, packs and splints*

- Allergic skin reactions.
- Ischaemia due to tight dressings.
- Cutaneous ulceration occurs particularly at knots, e.g. at the columella when a post-nasal pack is in place, and at the skin next to a knot when a tight head bandage is applied.
- Inhalation, particularly of nasal packs and splints.
- Delayed identification of wound infection.
- Failure to remove the dressings, e.g. aural dressings.

Complications of otological surgery

The specific complications are:

1. Reduction or loss of hearing.
2. Onset or exacerbation of tinnitus.
3. Onset or exacerbation of vertigo.
4. Onset or exacerbation of facial paralysis.
5. Haemorrhage.
6. CSF leak.
7. Meningitis.
8. Brain abscess.
9. External auditory canal stenosis.
10. Chronic aural discharge.
11. Aberrations of taste.

These complications may arise from poor surgical technique. However, they are more likely to occur for other reasons, which include:

1. Abnormal anatomy.
2. Extensive disease.
3. Failure of healing.
4. Post-operative infection.
5. Allergic reactions, e.g. to iodine in a pack.
6. No identifiable reason.

Methods of minimizing these complications are covered in Chapter 7.

Complications of nasal and sinus surgery

These are covered in Chapters 14, 15, 16, 17 and 18.

Complications of head and neck surgery

These are covered in Chapters 6, 7, 13, 19, 20, 21 and 22.

PRE-OPERATIVE INVESTIGATIONS

General

These will depend on the surgery planned and the general health of the patient.

1. Chest radiograph, ECG and respiratory function tests are required, particularly in smokers, the elderly and those with a history of cardiovascular or lung disease.
2. Full blood count.
3. Blood grouping, saving of serum and cross-matching of blood.
4. Urea and electrolytes and liver function tests.
5. Clotting studies if there is a history of a bleeding abnormality in the patient or family.

Otological

1. *Assessment of hearing*
    *   Pure tone audiogram with bone conduction.
    *   Free field audiogram, Kendal toy test or distraction testing may be necessary in young children. These tests often take a long time to perform and are not always available. If this is the situation then a clinical assessment of hearing should be made.
    *   A speech audiogram. This gives useful additional information, particularly if the pure tone audiogram is unreliable.

- Evoked response audiometry. This is rarely required purely as an investigation of hearing prior to surgery. However, it should be considered in patients who are unable to perform the subjective tests listed above.

2. *Assessment of middle ear function*

- Tympanometry.

3. *Assessment of balance*

   This is rarely required prior to middle ear surgery. It is usually part of the clinical examination.
   - Caloric testing.
   - Electronystagmography.

   These tests are usually part of the diagnostic work-up of unilateral hearing loss and balance disorders. Consequently the results should be available prior to surgery for conditions such as Meniere's disease.

4. *Radiography*

Nasal and sinus surgery

1. Radiology.
   - Plain films.
   - Computerized tomography scanning.
   - Magnetic resonance imaging scanning.
   - Angiography.
2. Air flow study. This is rarely performed routinely in this country but will undoubtedly undergo development in future years.
3. Endoscopic assessment.
4. Photographs prior to rhinoplasty surgery.

Head and neck surgery

1. Radiographic. This is usually performed to assess the size and extent of the lesion to be treated surgically and to delineate the anatomy.
   - Plain films.
   - Computerized tomography.
   - Magnetic resonance imaging.
   - Ultrasonic imaging.
   - Contrast radiography, e.g. sialography.
   - Digital vascular imaging. Dynamic studies are occasionally necessary.
   - Doppler flow studies of arterial flow.
   - Angiography.
   - Videofluoroscopy or cineradiography.
   - Diaphragmatic screening.
   - Therapeutic intraventional radiography.
2. Cytology and histology from fine needle aspiration biopsy.

3. Laryngography. This may include stroboscopy, electromyography and other dynamic tests of laryngeal function.

THE THEATRE TEAM

Successful safe surgery is a team effort orchestrated by the surgeon. It is essential that all personnel involved are present and know their role. The team can be sub-divided into its constituent parts.

The service team

1. Cleaning services.
2. Maintenance engineers for plumbing, air conditioning, piped gases and equipment.
3. Sterile supply department engaged in the cleaning of reusable equipment and the provision of sterile instruments and drapes.
4. Purchasing department engaged in the supply of new and replacement equipment and drugs.
5. Prevention of infection team engaged in the monitoring of the cleanliness of the theatres.

The anaesthetic team

This usually consists of an anaesthetist and an assistant. In addition there is a nurse to aid in the recovery of the patient following anaesthesia.

The operating team

1. Surgeon and assistants.
2. The scrub nurse.
3. The 'running' or 'floor' nurse. This nurse collects instruments and sutures. In conjunction with the scrub nurse, the floor nurse will keep a count of swabs, needles and instruments.
4. There is often a fourth nurse cleaning and tidying instruments prior to dispatch for re-sterilization or preparing for the next case.

Supporting services

Members of other departments may be required to provide support services during an operation. Some common examples are:

1. Pathologist. Frozen section analysis.
2. Radiologist, e.g. intra-operative screening, immediate post-operative chest radiograph.
3. Neurophysiologist/audiologist.

Chapter 2

Basic principles of technique

PRE-OPERATIVE CHECKS

The patient

1. The correct patient by name and number.
2. The patient is adequately starved.
3. The correct operation and side.
4. The consent form is signed and the medical records are present.
5. All appropriate investigations are present, e.g. radiographs and audiograms.

These facts should be checked by the nurse receiving the patient into the operating suite, not only on the written documents and patient's name tag but by asking the patient directly. The surgeon should also check these facts before commencing the surgery. Errors most frequently arise when the operating order of a list is changed and when there are patients with similar names on the list. Beware especially of twins on the same list or even in the same hospital.

Positioning of the patient

The purpose of correct positioning is:

1. To facilitate ease of operating.
2. To prevent complications.
3. To keep the patient comfortable.

1. Facilitation of operating

- The height, tilt and roll of the table should be adjustable, thus the site of surgery can be kept in the optimum position. A foot-down tilt is useful to reduce bleeding by increasing venous drainage from the head.

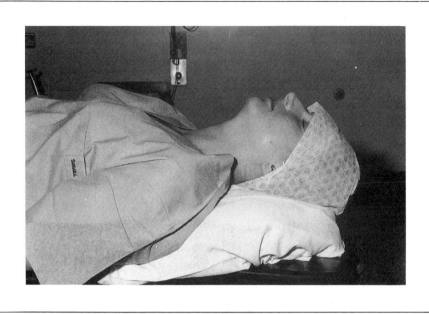

Figure 2.1 This is the 'sniffing morning air position' for endoscopy. The pillow is 'plumped' to achieve the optimal alignment for the insertion of the endosope. This system is very flexible

- The head section of the table should be adjustable to facilitate flexion and extension of the patient's neck (Figures 2.1 and 2.2).
- Sand bags or inflatable rubber bags can be used to stabilize the head in rotated positions, or under the shoulders to ease neck extension.
- Should the surgeon choose to sit, then an adjustable stool is an advantage. In microsurgery the operator should remember that the patient's position, the microscope's position and his or her own position are all flexible (Figure 2.3).
- The light source should be positionable.
- The scrub nurse and the surgeon's assistant should be positioned so they can work easily as a team without getting in each other's way.

2. Prevention of complications

The longer the operation the more likely that complications may arise as the result of suboptimal positioning.

- Attention should be paid to pressure areas. Moulded foam supports can be used to spread the load. Prolonged compression of the calves may lead to a risk of deep vein thrombosis; consequently pneumatic boots or support stockings may be required.

- If a large degree of roll is necessary there is always a risk that the patient may fall from the table – consequently retaining straps may be used. More likely, however, is the risk of an arm or leg falling off the table in an uncontrolled manner. Correctly positioned arm supports should prevent this problem.
- All mobile trolleys should have brakes.
- If surgery is likely to be prolonged it may be necessary to provide warmth. This can be done using a water blanket.
- If surgery is likely to be prolonged urinary catheterization may be necessary.

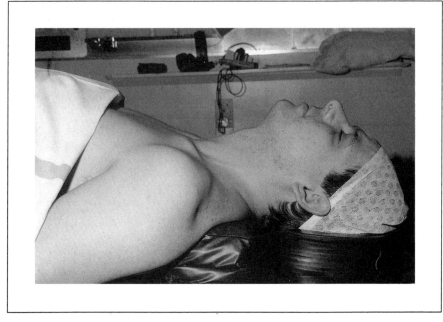

Figure 2.2 The patient positioned for neck surgery. The neck is extended and there is foot-down tilt of the table. The 'table break' is positioned between the sandbag under the shoulders and the head support. This permits a mechanism to increase the extension of the neck if it is required

THE SURGEON'S PREPARATION

Prior to scrubbing for surgery, the operator should take sensible steps. The operator should adjust the eye pieces on the operating microscope. If the surgeon wears glasses or eye protectors they should be clean. To prevent misting of glasses it may be necessary to tape the operating mask upper border to the cheeks. The headlight should be donned.

The hands and forearms should be scrubbed for 5 minutes using an anti-septic soap, paying particular attention to the nails. It is not necessary to use a scrubbing brush between cases. Gown and gloves should be donned using an aseptic technique. Any powder should be washed from the gloves using sterile water.

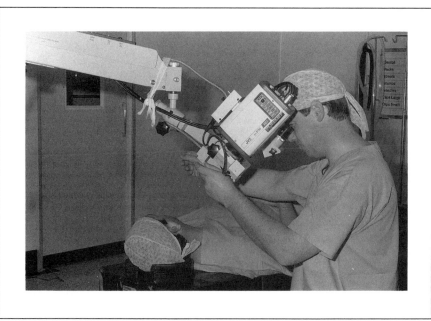

Figure 2.3   This is a patient positioned (but not skin prepared or draped) for mastoid surgery. The surgeon is placing the microscope in position. Note that his right hand is extended to where the operating assistant would give the instruments. The eyes should not leave the microscope as the surgeon is handed instruments

THE PATIENT'S PREPARATION

On the ward

1. The patient should have a bath and hair wash.
2. All items of jewellery, false teeth and other prostheses should be removed and retained on the ward. In jaw surgery the false teeth may be required in the operating room. In this circumstance they should accompany the patient.
3. The site of operation should be shaved and any loose hair cleaned from the skin. The eyebrows should never be shaved. It may be necessary to take a separate written consent when a head shave is required, especially in a woman.
4. The patient should go to the toilet.
5. The teeth should be cleaned.
6. The patient should be dressed in a clean operating gown. The patient may wear a personal pair of clean underpants except when surgery on the

abdomen or thighs is contemplated, when disposable underwear should be worn. A child should be allowed to bring a favourite toy or 'soothing' blanket to theatre. This should not be brought into the operating room but taken direct from the anaesthetic room to the recovery area ready for the child when they wake.

In theatre

1. Prior to placing sterile drapes on the patient the following should occur:
   - The patient should be positioned.
   - Diathermy pad should be attached.
   - Monitoring equipment should be attached.
   - The skin should be cleaned. An antiseptic preparation should be used to clean the skin. When this contains alcohol the excess should be wiped off to reduce the risks of fire when diathermy is used. Many surgeons prefer not to use any preparation in the external auditory canal because of the risk of ototoxic damage.
   - Any necessary protective packing should be placed, e.g. throat packs.
2. The patient is draped. The drapes should be secured with clips or adhesive tape. It may be necessary to suture the drapes to the skin. Suction tubing is clipped to the drapes. The diathermy lead is clipped to the drapes, taking care not to damage the cable insulation. A quiver is clipped to the drapes to hold the diathermy forceps.

DIATHERMY

Unipolar

The patient is part of the electrical circuit. Heat is generated at the point where the maximum amount of electrical current is passing through a small volume of tissue. In normal working conditions this is the point where the forceps or needle are in contact with the patient when the operating pedal is pushed and the circuit is closed. Bearing this principle in mind, diathermy should not be used on tissue attached to the patient by a pedicle. The neutral plate must be in contact with a large area of skin, otherwise a burn can occur at the point of contact. The diathermy forceps should be kept in a quiver lest a burn result through accidental pressing of the operating pedal. Great care should be taken if the diathermy current is being applied through non-insulated instruments. A burn will result at every point that the instrument comes in contact with the patient.

The cutting mode is useful for cutting across muscle. A blend of cutting and coagulation will give less bleeding when cutting muscle.

If the machine 'alarms' (Figure 2.4) then the following points should be checked:

1. The patient is not earthed through the metal of the operating table.

2.   The diathermy lead and the neutral plates are connected to the machine.
3.   The neutral plate is connected to the patient.

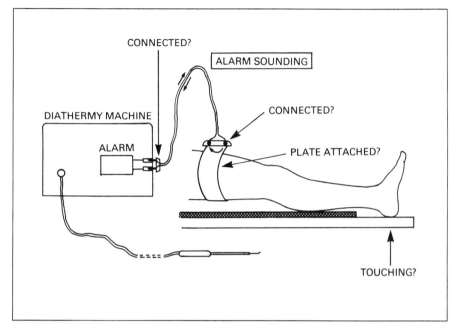

Figure 2.4   A unipolar diathermy circuit (from OGS, by permission)

Bipolar

In this circumstance the current is conducted between the tips of the forceps. This tool is useful for obtaining a fine controlled burn. In use the forceps are held with the tips slightly apart. The tissue between the tips is then heated. It is safe to use bipolar diathermy on pedicles and close to structures that are delicate. It is of particular use in resection of skull base tumours such as acoustic neuromas and in parotidectomy.

THE OPERATING MICROSCOPE

This is arguably the most important tool of the modern ENT surgeon, who should be familiar with its use in the temporal bone laboratory. The appropriate objective lenses to achieve the optimal working distance are, for ear work, a 200 mm or 250 mm lens, for sinus surgery a 300 mm lens and for microlaryngeal work a 400 mm lens. The surgeon should know their correct setting for the eye pieces. Most microscopes have a greenish filter which will highlight blood vessels by making them appear black.

OTHER SPECIAL EQUIPMENT

Drills and power saws

These have either rotating or oscillating cutting heads. The otologist's drill is dealt with in Chapter 7. Care should be taken that they only come into contact with bone that requires cutting. The oscillating saw will do less damage to soft tissues than the rotating type. Where possible a guard should be used on the saw. Training should be sought before using these tools for the first time. These tools throw off a fine mist of blood and bone. To reduce the risk of contracting a blood-borne infection through the conjunctivae, safety glasses should be worn.

Nerve stimulators

A simple disposable nerve stimulator can be very helpful in identifying the facial nerve during middle ear and parotid surgery, especially in situations where the anatomy has been distorted by the disease process. The passive electrode is placed into muscle and the active electrode is used to stimulate.

In intra-cranial surgery on the facial nerve intra-operative electrophysiological monitoring is helpful in identification of the nerve. Neurogenic recording electrodes can be placed on the face. These are connected to an audible and visible monitor. A nerve stimulator with a variable output can be used to identify the nerve. An increase in latency of the evoked action potential of the nerve or a decrease in its amplitude can alert the surgeon to damage by manipulation during surgery; for example, at removal of an acoustic neuroma.

Eighth nerve monitoring

Click-generated sound is delivered to the test ear via an ear mould. Transtympanic or external auditory canal electrodes record the compound eighth nerve action potential and the auditory brainstem responses intra-operatively. A fine silver electrode can be used to record direct from the cochlear nerve, hence the cochlear nerve can be identified during surgery for acoustic neuroma and vestibular neurectomy.

The carbon dioxide laser

Stimulated emission of infra-red radiation from CO_2 molecules in a carbon dioxide, nitrogen and helium gas mixture is powered by an electrical discharge through the gas. The gaseous lasing medium is held in a resonant cavity between two mirrors. One of the mirrors is semi-transparent so that a continuous infra-red beam can exit. The light beam is parallel, coherent and monochromatic. There is no suitable fibre-optic delivery system. The CO_2 laser used in ENT practice has an invisible working beam that comes to a focal point at 400 mm from the aperture of the instrument.

The neodynium–YAG laser

The rare earth neodynium is incorporated into the crystalline lattice of yttrium aluminium garnet to produce a material of sufficient strength to withstand the impact of continuous laser light. The wavelength of the light produced is close to the infra-red end of the spectrum. This gives the Nd–YAG laser the greatest penetrating power of all commercially available medical lasers.

This laser light can pass through optical fibre, consequently the tool may be used in a flexible fibre-optic endoscope. The tip of the fibre is kept clean by directing a stream of carbon dioxide gas over the tip. A helium–neon laser is incorporated into the path of the Nd–YAG laser to provide a visible aiming beam. As an endoscopic attachment its main use by the ENT surgeon is in the management of tracheal stenosis. As a hand-held tool the Nd–YAG laser may also be used as a 'knife'.

Safety precautions with medical lasers

The hazards to patients and staff are:

1. Corneal injury with the CO_2 laser and retinal damage with the Nd–YAG laser.
2. Unintentional burns to the patient or staff.
3. Combustion, explosion or toxic gas production if the beam impinges on undesired material.
4. Reflections from reflective material in the infra-red spectrum extend all the above hazards beyond the immediate operative area.

(Reference: The reader is advised to consult Oswal, V. H., Flood, L. F and Kashima, H (1988) *The CO_2 Laser in Otolaryngology and Head and Neck Surgery*, Wright, London)

A summary of safety precautions is:

1. The laser should only be used in a 'laser controlled area'.
2. Laser warning signs should be placed outside the theatre and next to the exit port on the laser.
3. The laser should be well maintained. Before use it should be tested and the alignment of the aiming laser beam checked.
4. The working area should be protected, especially the patient's face and eyes. The patient must be protected. Moist protection should be used with the CO_2 laser.
5. Adequate suction should be used to aspirate the smoke and vaporized tissue.
6. Suitable protection for the eyes of all staff and the patient should be used. These include protection goggles and attenuation filters in endoscopic laser surgery.
7. Matt instruments to minimize reflection.
8. Special endotracheal tubes.
9. Oxygen/nitrous oxide mixture should not be used for inhalation anaesthesia. Nitrous oxide supports combustion.

10. Only properly trained and approved surgeons, anaesthetists and nursing staff should perform the surgery.

PATHOLOGICAL SPECIMENS FROM THE OPERATING ROOM

All specimens must be correctly labelled with:

1. The name, age, hospital number and ward of the patient.
2. The name of the surgeon in charge.
3. Type and source of specimen.
4. The laboratory to which the specimen is to be sent.

It is usual for an accompanying request form to be sent which must give the patient's history and clinical findings. There is often much to be gained by discussing the patient with the pathologist in advance of 'taking' a specimen. In this way the laboratory can say how they require the material, e.g. fresh, in formalin, and whether they require other biopsies as well, e.g. blood, bone marrow, brushings for cytology.

Histology

Routinely specimens are sent in formalin. However, when a reticuloendo-thelial tumour is suspected fresh material is often required. It is important that when fresh material is to be sent that it is dispatched promptly and that the laboratory is warned in advance. Fresh epithelium is required for ciliary motility studies.

Electron microscopy requires special fixatives. These should be requested in advance. Formalin fixation is not suitable.

Orientation of the specimen is often difficult for the pathologist. If this is important, as in a neck dissection, the specimen should be pinned out on a sheet of cork and labelled. Alternatively, 'marking sutures' of different lengths or colours should be placed at critical spots to help orientation of the specimen. These marking sutures are listed on the request form. After biopsy of an unusual lesion it is wise to send a fresh specimen in transport medium to the bacteriology laboratory.

Bacteriology

Swabs are routinely placed in transport medium before being dispatched to the laboratory. Dry swabs should not be used routinely except when it can be guaranteed that they will reach the laboratory within two hours. Fungal and TB culture must be specifically requested as these are not routine procedures.

All specimens should reach the laboratory within a few hours. Pus swabs in transport medium can be kept in a refrigerator overnight, as can urine specimens. Fresh pus must always be sent direct to the laboratory for immediate attention. Blood cultures need to be placed in an incubator as soon as possible after preparation.

Virology studies should be discussed with the laboratory concerned.

POST-OPERATIVE CHECKS IN THE OPERATING ROOM

Prior to closure of the patient's wound the scrub nurse should:

1. Perform an instrument count and check that none of the instruments has been damaged.
2. Perform a swab count.
3. Perform a needle count.

If anything is missing then a thorough search should be made, including a radiological investigation if necessary. This will usually trace the missing item. If anything is still missing after a further diligent search inside the patient, the patient's wound should be closed.

At the end of the operation the scrub nurse should do a further:

1. Instrument count and check.
2. Swab count, especially pledgets, woolly balls and patties.
3. Needle count.
4. Make a note of everything that has been deliberately left in the patient, including the nature of the dressings. The batch number and code number of any implants should be recorded.

Once the surgeon has been informed that all these checks are in order the operator may assist the anaesthetist to recover the patient.

It is important that the anaesthetist:

1. Accounts for all anaesthetic swabs, needles and glass vials.
2. Checks that the endotracheal tube is intact.
3. Ensures that all oral packing has been removed.
4. Checks that the teeth are undamaged.

Should any item still be unaccounted for at this stage then the following procedures should be adopted:

1. As each drape is removed from the patient it is thoroughly examined.
2. The surgeon, assistant and the scrub nurse, one at a time, step away from the table onto a green towel laid on the floor. Each shakes carefully over the towel, then carefully disrobes. The operating gowns are all thoroughly examined.
3. The instrument trolley is thoroughly examined, especially unused swabs and folded drapes. The instruments are individually counted off the trolley.
4. The soles of the shoes of every person who was in the theatre are examined before they leave the theatre, as are the inside of surgeons' boots.

5.   The patient is very thoroughly examined, as are the blankets and clothes, before the patient is wheeled to the recovery room.
6.   The operating table and anaesthetic machine are moved, then the room is thoroughly swept.
7.   All these actions and their outcome are noted in the patient's records.

If the item is still missing and it is known to be radio-opaque appropriate radiographs should be taken once the patient has recovered from the anaesthetic.

WRITING THE OPERATION RECORD

The operation notes consist of two parts: the anaesthetic record and the surgery record.

The anaesthetic record

This should record the following information:

1.   The pre-medication.
2.   Method of induction.
3.   Details of ventilation.
4.   Details of intubation.
5.   Monitoring methods.
6.   Site and nature of vascular access.
7.   History of the anaesthetic including blood pressure readings, infusions and drugs given.
8.   Additional equipment used, e.g. water blanket, catheterization and rectal thermometer.
9.   Recovery of the patient.
10. Instructions concerning post-operative care and analgesia.

The surgical record

This should record the following information:

1.   Name of the surgeon and any assistants. Should anything unexpected arise during the surgery that may mitigate against an optimal outcome then the names of any other individual to whom this was demonstrated should be recorded. Furthermore, if convenient, photographs should be taken of any unexpected finding.
2.   A description of the incision.
3.   The surgical approach to reach the pathology should be described.
4.   A description of the pathological findings.
5.   The method by which the pathology was treated.
6.   A description of all biopsies and specimens sent for analysis.

7. Any implants left in the patient should be noted with any batch or code numbers.
8. Closure of the wound.
9. Details for further management, e.g. when sutures and dressings should be removed.
10. The expected outcome of the surgery.
11. Any difficult or unexpected circumstances:
    - Bleeding.
    - Unusual anatomical variations.
    - Technical problems with equipment.
    - Unexpected pathology.

After surgery the operator should inform the patient as to the success of the operation.

Chapter 3

Anaesthesia

LOCAL ANAESTHESIA

Myringotomy

Two or three metered doses of 10% lignocaine aerosol spray are directed towards the upper wall of the auditory canal and the solution is allowed to run down over the tympanic membrane. After about 5 minutes the procedure may be performed. The degree of anaesthesia is poor.

A eutectic mixture of local anaesthesia EMLA (trade name) cream may be used as it has a better penetrating power. This cream is applied carefully to the tympanic membrane at the proposed site of myringotomy. After 20 to 30 minutes the cream is aspirated and a myringotomy and even grommet insertion may be performed.

Mastoidectomy and tympanotomy

Approximately 10–15 ml of 0.5–1% lignocaine with 1:200 000 adrenaline is used in total. Between 1 and 3 ml are injected at each site.

The greater auricular nerve is blocked by injecting a number of sites over the mastoid process (Figure 3.1). The main nerve trunk may also be blocked by injecting approximately 2.5 cm below the mastoid at the anterior border of sternomastoid.

The auricular branch of the vagus is blocked by injecting into the skin of the floor of the auditory canal and periosteally on the anterior surface of the mastoid process.

The auriculotemporal nerve is anaesthetized by injecting between the bony and cartilaginous parts of the anterior aspect of the external auditory canal. The skin and periosteum over the root of the zygoma should also be infiltrated (Figure 3.2).

A few drops of 4% lignocaine can be instilled into the middle ear cleft to obtain anaesthesia of the mucous membrane.

A facial paralysis is usual with this technique. This palsy recovers after a few hours. For a tympanotomy, blocking the auriculotemporal nerve and its tympanic branch is often all that is necessary.

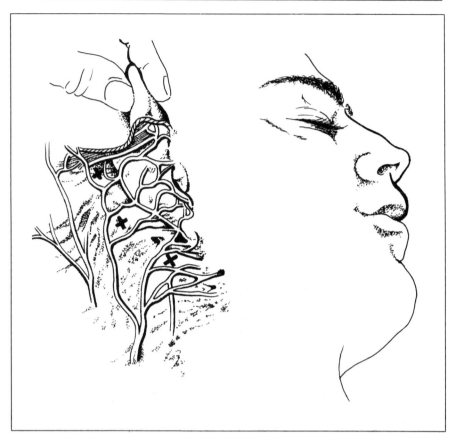

Figure 3.1 The crosses denote the sites of injection to block the greater auricular nerve over the mastoid process and highlights the ramifications of the nerve. This demonstrates the need for wide infiltration

Should the patient experience nausea during the procedure this may be abolished by the intravenous injection of 1% lignocaine in a dose of 1 mg/kg body weight.

Operations on the nose and septum

To anaesthetize the external nose, a needle is passed superiorly between the upper and lower lateral cartilages upwards to the glabella. Alternatively, the skin is penetrated at the glabella and the needle passed down to the alae nasi. Lignocaine 1% with 1:200 000 adrenaline is injected as the needle is withdrawn. The external lateral wall of the nose is anaesthetized by four passes of the needle from the glabella laterally (Figure 3.3).

The bases of the alae nasi are anaesthetized by direct infiltration. From within the nostril the needle is passed close to the periosteum along the line of the planned lateral osteotomies and the area infiltrated.

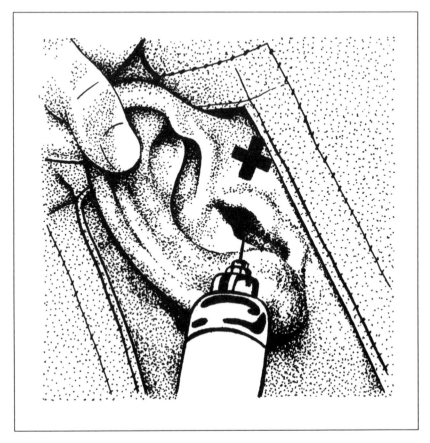

Figure 3.2 Sites of injection to block the auriculotemporal nerve

Local anaesthetic is infiltrated at the sites of the intra-cartilaginous incisions and posterior to the columella. The base of the columella must be anaesthetized.

About 5–8 ml solution of lignocaine 1% with 1:200 000 adrenaline is used to numb the external nose.

The internal nose may be anaesthetized by packing the cavity with gauze soaked in cocaine and adrenaline solution. No more than 3 mg/kg of cocaine should be administered. Alternatively, lignocaine 4% can be used. The pack should be left in place for about 20 minutes.

A sub-perichondral injection of 1% lignocaine with 1:200 000 adrenaline into the septum will give reasonable anaesthesia as well as facilitate septal dissection.

Maxillary antral puncture

Four per cent lignocaine is sprayed into the nose. Cotton wool wrapped onto malleable wires is soaked in 10% cocaine solution and placed under the inferior

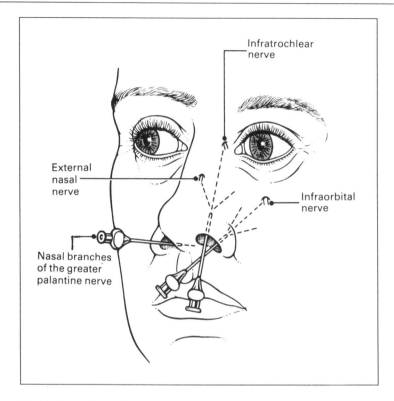

Figure 3.3 Injection technique for local anaesthesia in nasal surgery (from RSN, by permission)

turbinate. The cotton wool is left in place for 20 minutes, then the puncture performed.

Caldwell–Luc operation

The gingiva are sprayed with 4% lignocaine. The nasal cavity on the side of the operation is anaesthetized with ribbon gauze soaked in cocaine solution (approximately 100 mg of cocaine is used for an adult). The sublabial soft tissues are infiltrated with 1% lignocaine with 1:100 000 adrenaline. When the maxillary antrum is opened, cocaine-soaked ribbon gauze is inserted.

Laryngoscopy and bronchoscopy

The oropharynx is sprayed with 4% lignocaine. In the edentulous patient the upper gingiva must be anaesthetized. An injection of 0.5% lignocaine is effective. Next a laryngeal spray loaded with 4% lignocaine is used to anaesthetize the larynx. This should be done during intonation (Figure 3.4). The solution should be allowed to run down into the trachea. The trachea can be directly anaesthetized by injecting 1–2 ml of 2% lignocaine through the mid line of the cricothyroid membrane.

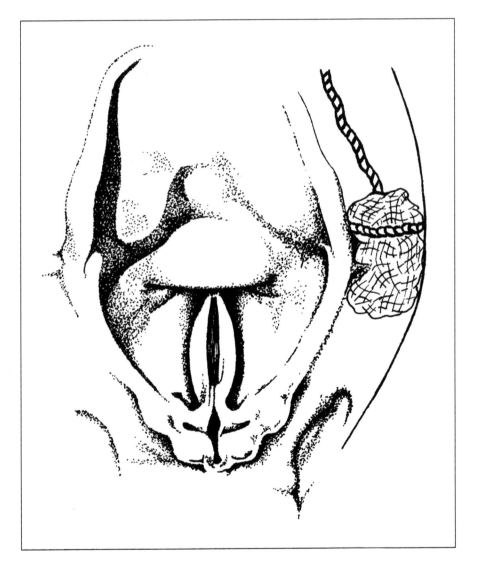

Figure 3.4 A pack soaked in cocaine solution has been placed in the pyriform fossa to anaesthetize the submucosal superior laryngeal nerve. This achieves anaesthesia of the supraglottic hemilarynx prior to endoscopy

Great care should be taken to monitor the total dose of lignocaine delivered. The maximum is 3 mg/kg body weight, although this value can increase if the lignocaine is combined with adrenaline.

Fibre-optic bronchoscopy

The larger nasal passage is chosen and sprayed three times with 10% lignocaine, giving 10 mg/spray. The scope is lubricated with lignocaine gel. The oropharynx may be sprayed. Oxygen is delivered via a fine catheter inserted through the other nostril which has been previously anaesthetized.

When the scope reaches the epiglottis, four 0.5 ml aliquots of lignocaine 1% are injected through the scope. After a few minutes the scope is passed through the larynx. During the progression of the scope further aliquots are given as necessary. A total dose of 3 mg/kg should not be exceeded.

Tonsillectomy

The tonsil area is innervated by branches from the glossopharyngeal nerve as it passes down the stylopharyngeal muscle.

Lignocaine 4% spray is used to anaesthetize the oropharyngeal mucous membrane. Ten to fifteen ml of 0.5% lignocaine with 1:200 000 adrenaline is administered on each side. The posterior palatal arch is infiltrated first. The tonsil is then pulled medially to help demarcate the capsule. The anterior arch is then infiltrated. The tongue is depressed and the base of the tonsil and the tonsillar attachment are injected.

Tracheostomy

Cutaneous and deep tissue infiltration with 1% lignocaine with 1:200 000 adrenaline is usually adequate. Some local anaesthetic should be injected into the trachea prior to creation of the formal opening.

Indications for local anaesthesia

1. When general anaesthesia is contra-indicated.
2. When the patient expresses a preference for local anaesthesia.
3. Tympanotomy, stapedectomy and tympanoplasty when there is an advantage in having the patient awake and hearing.
4. Ultrasonic and cryotherapeutic destruction of the labyrinth.
5. Microlaryngoscopy when there is an advantage in having the patient awake and phonating, e.g. when administering a Teflon paste injection.

Contra-indications for local anaesthesia

1. Children under the age of 16.
2. Nervous individuals.
3. Those who express a preference for general anaesthesia.
4. Lignocaine allergy.

5. Adrenaline should be used with great caution in patients:
   - suffering from thyrotoxicosis, hypertension or ischaemic heart disease;
   - under general anaesthesia when halothane, trichloroethylene or cyclo-propane is being administered;
   - receiving tricyclic antidepressants.

Pre-medication for local anaesthesia

This should be carefully tailored to the individual. Morphine or papaveretum with a phenothiazine is a popular combination because of the amnesia and sense of euphoria induced. Anxiety in theatre can be controlled by intravenous benzodiazepines, such as Diazemuls or midazolam.

GENERAL ANAESTHESIA

Anaesthesia for post-tonsillectomy bleeding

It is vitally important that experienced personnel deal with this emergency. A junior anaesthetist assisting a junior surgeon to operate on a shocked bleeding child is a recipe for disaster. Firstly, an intravenous line should be placed and the child resuscitated. Cross-matched blood should be available, but if the child is deteriorating rapidly due to blood loss and a plasma expander is inadequate it is permissible to give uncross-matched blood. Central depressants should be avoided to quieten a restless bleeding child unless the child can be closely supervised.

Anaesthetic induction should not be commenced until the patient is on an adjustable operating table and running suction is available.

If the oropharynx is clear of blood, anaesthesia can be induced in a head-up supine position using isofluorane with a curare-like muscle relaxant. Nasal intubation should be avoided as this may precipitate further haemorrhage. Suxamethonium is best avoided as the drug raises intra-gastric pressure with the consequent risk of vomiting.

When bleeding is brisk, anaesthesia can be induced in a head-down, right lateral position. The staff should be prepared to cope with gastric regurgitation. Intubation is possible, but can be difficult. Alternatively, once deep anaesthesia has been induced the Boyle–Davis gag can be inserted and intubation avoided. The patient is then turned into the tonsillectomy position whilst suction is used to keep the pharynx clear and the bleeding controlled.

Vomiting in recovery must be expected. Most anaesthetists prefer to aspirate the stomach via a Ryle's tube prior to recovery.

Anaesthesia in rigid bronchoscopy

In rigid oesophagoscopy there is little problem for the anaesthetist as the airway can be secured with tracheal intubation. However, bronchoscopy requires close co-operation between the surgeon and anaesthetist because they must share the airway. There are three basic techniques.

1. Spontaneous respiration

Spontaneous respiration is essential in a patient with copious secretions, inhaled foreign bodies, bronchial–pleural fistulae and lung bullae. It is also an advantage in very young children where short periods of apnoea may lead to severe hypoxaemia. When combined with local anaesthesia, conditions are usually adequate for minor procedures. Sufficient relaxation may be difficult to achieve in an adult.

2. Oxygen insufflation with apnoea and anaesthesia

Up to 20 minutes' operating time can be achieved with complete surgical relaxation by using intravenous anaesthesia with a muscle relaxant. Oxygen is supplied to the trachea via a fine catheter at a rate of 6–10 litres/min. With the use of this technique there is a steady rise in alveolar PCO_2.

3. Venturi type positive pressure insufflation with apnoea and anaesthesia

This is similar to the insufflation technique described above, except that oxygen is intermittently injected under high pressure via the bronchoscope. Adequate ventilation can be provided for an almost indefinite period of time in the relaxed, apnoeic patient.

General anaesthesia for microlaryngoscopy

Not only must the surgeon and anaesthetist share the airway but the surgeon's vision may be hampered by a large anaesthetic tube.

1. General anaesthesia with spontaneous respiration

Anaesthesia is induced with an intravenous agent. A depth of anaesthesia is obtained using nitrous oxide, oxygen and isofluorane to provide relaxation. The larynx and pharynx are sprayed with topical anaesthetic. A 3 mm plastic tube is inserted via the nose as far as the lower trachea, through which oxygen is blown at 12–15 litres/min. Anaesthesia is maintained using intravenous fentanyl. This gives a good view to the surgeon.

2. Intubation

A 5 mm cuffed nasotracheal tube gives perfect airway protection, and provided hand ventilation through a circle absorber is used, adequate respiratory exchange for up to 45 minutes. This gives a reasonable view for the surgeon in the adult patient.

3. Positive pressure ventilation using a Venturi injector

The Carden laryngoscopy tube is placed below the larynx and the cuff inflated. A similar technique to that in bronchoscopy is used for anaesthesia. This gives an excellent view to the surgeon.

Anaesthesia for upper respiratory obstruction

The anaesthetist should never be coerced into attempting to give a general anaesthetic against better judgement. Where the risk is great it is always preferable to perform the procedure under local anaesthesia.

A partial airway obstruction can rapidly be converted to a total obstruction when the patient is rendered unconscious. Therefore the following preparations are essential before attempting to deliver a general anaesthetic in a patient with respiratory obstruction:

1. No narcotics prior to induction.
2. Avoid atropine. It increases brain oxygen requirements and makes secretions more tenacious.
3. The surgical team should be gloved and ready lest an emergency arise.
4. The patient should be pre-oxygenated. Heliox is useful for this.
5. In cases of significant obstruction an inhalation induction should be used to achieve a depth of relaxation prior to attempting intubation.

If intubation is impossible then a tracheostomy should be performed immediately.

Any operation on the obstructed infant larynx should be preceded by a tracheostomy. In major surgery on the pharynx, oral cavity and tongue, the possibility of obstruction due to post-operative oedema should be borne in mind. It is frequently wiser to perform a tracheostomy at the start of such surgery.

Obtaining the bloodless field in ENT surgery

Bleeding at the site of surgery depends on:

1. The venous pressure at the operation field.
2. Peripheral arteriolar circulation.

Venous ooze can be kept to a minimum by:

1. Correct posture. In ENT surgery this usually means a (head-up) tilt on the operating table.
2. Careful anaesthetic technique to minimize coughing and straining.
3. Maintenance of an adequate airway.

Reduction of peripheral arteriolar circulation may be achieved by:

1. Local vasoconstrictor drugs.
2. Hypotensive anaesthetic techniques.

Hypotensive anaesthesia

A thorough cardiovascular examination and drug history are essential with ECG, chest X-ray, full blood count and sickle cell test when appropriate.

Myocardial ischaemia and cerebrovascular insufficiency are absolute contra-indications.

Hypotension is best avoided in:

1. Hypertensive patients on drug therapy.
2. Diabetic patients who are unstable when given ganglion blockers.
3. Pregnancy.
4. Anaemia or other blood dyscrasias.
5. Hypo- and hyperthyroid states.
6. Patients on the contraceptive pill.

The anaesthetist tries to achieve a dry operating field by reducing the systolic blood pressure to about 65 mmHg. This is done by lowering the cardiac output and decreasing the peripheral resistance while maintaining adequate tissue perfusion. Levels below 55 mmHg at arm level run the risk of cerebral ischaemia.

The cardiac output is reduced by:

1. Pooling blood in the lower extremities by posture and muscle relaxation.
2. Using isofluorane or halothane to reduce myocardial contractile force.
3. Using a beta blocker to reduce contractile force and heart rate.

The peripheral resistance may be reduced by:

1. Central depression of the vasomotor centre with isofluorane or halothane.
2. Ganglion blockade.
3. Peripheral vasodilation with sodium nitroprusside.

Monitoring of the patient with ECG and blood pressure monitoring is vital during the procedure (Figure 3.5). In prolonged procedures an intra-arterial line for blood pressure monitoring may be required. In major surgery with significant blood loss, monitoring of central venous pressure may be required. In prolonged surgery monitoring of the temperature may be required.

THE ROLE OF THE SURGEON IN PREVENTING ANAESTHETIC ACCIDENTS

Mutual respect and close co-operation between the anaesthetist and the surgeon are essential. At no time should the surgeon try to prevail over the anaesthetist's better judgement when it comes to matters relating to the delivery of a safe anaesthetic. However, the vigilance of both during an operation may spot potential accidents. Potential hazards that the surgeon is in a particular position to observe include:

1. Failure to remove oral and pharyngeal packs prior to anaesthetic recovery.

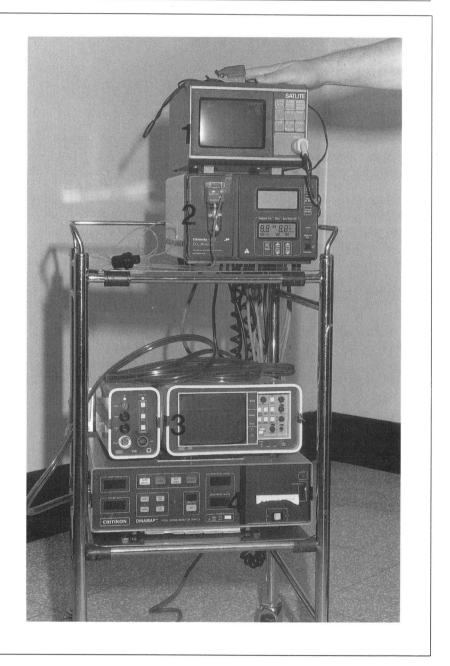

Figure 3.5 Anaesthetic monitors are shown on this trolley: 1. Pulse oximeter (finger attachment on top of machine); 2. CO_2 monitor; 3. ECG machine; 4. Dinamap blood pressure monitor

2. A change in the colour of the patient.
3. A change in the colour of the patient's blood.

4. Developing oedema in the upper airways that might necessitate securing the airway by tracheostomy prior to completion of the surgical procedure.
5. Warning the anaesthetist of the intention to open the larynx or trachea well in advance in major neck surgery.
6. Failure of respiration (this might occur should the anaesthetic delivery system become disconnected).
7. Warning the anaesthetist of the intention of giving certain drugs such as cocaine or adrenaline.

In procedures in which the airway is shared the surgeon must give the anaesthetist an explanation of the proposed surgery and its likely duration.

Although it is the anaesthetist's responsibility to assess the patient's fitness for anaesthesia not every patient will report all relevant facts. Should the surgeon be aware of any information that might make the operation out of the ordinary, e.g. a family history of anaesthetic problems, then it is as well to mention it to the anaesthetist. In this way an accident might be prevented and most anaesthetists rarely resent this incursion into their area of responsibility.

Chapter 4

Reconstructive materials in otolaryngology

Many substances are used in surgical practice to reconstruct, replace or augment the physiological or anatomical features of natural body tissues in the ear, nose or throat. These reconstructive substances can be organic or inorganic.

Organic substances are considered grafts whereas inorganic substances are termed biomaterials. Suture material will not be considered in this section.

GRAFTS

1. An *autograft* is when the donor and the recipient are the same person. Examples of autografts would include an incus transposition to reconstruct the ossicular chain, the use of sculpted septal cartilage to reconstruct the ossicular chain, or the use of bone grafts from either the ribs or the iliac crest to reconstruct the nose.
2. An *allograft* is when the donor and recipient are different individuals of the same species. A homograft is an allograft in a human individual. Most allografts have to be treated in some way to reduce the antigenicity of the implant and to reduce the incidence of tissue rejection. The potential transmission of disease (HIV virus, Creutzfeldt–Jakob) through an implanted allograft has reduced considerably the use of these materials. Examples of allografts used in otolaryngology prior to the AIDS epidemic were incus allografts, the use of lyophilized dura to repair tympanic membrane defects, and total middle ear allografts. Most of these allografts were stored in 70% alcohol.
3. A *heterograft* or a *xenograft* is when the donor and recipient are of different species. There are hardly any examples of xenografts designed as permanent implants in current otolaryngological practice, although there are a number of examples of temporary heterografts. Pig skin is sometimes used as a temporary dressing in cases of cutaneous thermal burns, and in otology absorbable alginate dressings derived from seaweed are very commonly used for support in the middle ear.

BIOMATERIALS

Biomaterials are synthetic or treated materials used to replace or augment tissues and organs. Inorganic implants are usually formed from one of three materials – plastics, metals, or ceramics. The term *'alloplastic implant'* can be used to describe an inorganic implant; however, this term does not imply that the implant is plastic. Alloplastic material (biomaterials) have always been of particular interest to the otologist concerned with middle ear reconstruction. The ideal biomaterial for implantation requires a number of qualities:

1. The material should not be rejected by the host.
2. The host should not require medication to prevent rejection.
3. The material should integrate with the host tissues.
4. The material should maintain its shape and structure, and therefore continue to function effectively throughout the lifetime of the patient.
5. The material should be easy to work with and be easily shaped surgically to an individual patient's need.
6. There should be no risk of transmission of any form of infection.
7. There should be no risk of carcinogenesis.
8. The ideal material should be inexpensive and widely available.
9. Thorough animal studies and controlled patient studies should be performed before a new biomaterial is extensively advertised and used.

There is no ideal biomaterial and most substances have a number of drawbacks. Typically, a new biomaterial appears on the scene and it is heralded in the initial published literature as being almost ideal. There follows an explosion in the use of the new material. Subsequently, the drawbacks of the material become apparent and new literature carries a number of reports concerning the disadvantages of the material. Sometimes the drawbacks are so severe that the material ceases to be used, or more commonly the material is used for a small number of specific indications by a small band of experts. Occasionally, the implant and the associated surgical technique are highly successful although examples of this situation are far out-numbered by the unsuccessful implants and surgical techniques. Examples of success stories include the alloplastic implant to replace the stapes in the operation of stapedectomy for otosclerosis, the osseointegrated screw of Brånemark, and the artificial hip replacement of Charnley.

The recent developments in biomaterial science have resulted in a revival in the use of middle ear alloplastic prostheses. These newer materials are also being used as implants in maxillofacial surgery for reconstruction of bony defects and in rhinology for nasal augmentation and repair of septal perforations. The selection of a particular material for reconstructive surgery is based on a number of factors which include physical, chemical, biochemical and surgical requirements. Some of these characteristics will be considered below.

1. Biocompatibility

Biocompatibility is the interaction between an implant and the body. Ideally this must lead to good and permanent integration of the prosthesis without degradation or rejection of the prosthesis and consequent loss of reconstructive function. This successful integration is dependent on the interface between the body and the surface of the implant material.

An implant material is *bioinert* if the body does not react to the substance. It is *biotolerant* if the body reacts to the implant material as if to a foreign body, but, after incorporation ceases to react to the implant. The material is *bioactive* if the body has an active surface compatibility with the alloplastic material which results in firm integration between the body and the foreign material.

Since the implant material is always placed in a wound, normal wound reactions to a foreign body inevitably occur. A bioinert material will be encapsulated by a small fibrous capsule. A biotolerant material will have a good fibrous capsule around the implant, often with giant cells present for many years. A bioactive material will develop a firm bond between the implant material and the body without an apparent capsule.

2.   Biomaterial structure

Formerly most implant materials were solid. In the last few years, however, porous materials have been developed which enable the host tissue to grow into the porous part of the implant with the hope that this would improve integration into the body. It has been found that micropores of approximately 100 micrometres were ideal for the ingrowth of fibrous tissue. Micropores facilitate the resorption and remodelling in living tissue but can be a problem in those materials which are not intended to degrade.

3.   Biodegradation

Practically all biomaterials will be affected by the body and some resorption will take place. The larger the surface area of the implant the greater the response by the body. Corrosion of metal implants can result in the release of potentially harmful substances such as nickel, colbalt, chromium and aluminium. This may result in allergic responses. Polymers can undergo degradation and on occasion some of the resultant substances can be very toxic. Ceramics may release substances into the body.

One particularly serious consequence of the materials released by biodegradation is the potential carcinogenic property of these substances. This has been demonstrated in animal experiments for some of the polymers, but has not been reported from clinical studies.

Bacteria are attracted to foreign bodies (such as an implant) within a wound. On occasion it may be impossible to remove a wound infection in the presence of an implant.

MATERIALS FOR IMPLANT

Prior to insertion of an implant one should check the precise nature of the compound, its biocompatibility and its integration capacity in surgical application. Some products only have the trade names and this can be particularly unhelpful. The three main types of biomaterial used in otolaryngology are metals, polymers and ceramics.

1. Metals

Metals are not commonly used in otolaryngology and most of the long-term clinical experience comes from orthopaedics. Most metal implants would cause considerable infection risk and result in a marked wound reaction, with the exception of gold, silver and platinum. The applications of gold and silver are restricted by the softness of these two metals.

There are a large number of alloy steels with variable resistance to corrosion. None is perfect. There are three particular classes of alloys used in medical reconstruction. These are:

- The cobalt chromium group.
- The stainless steel group.
- The titanium group.

The cobalt chromium alloy group is particularly useful. Vitalium is the most frequently used trade name. These alloys are widely used in the fields of orthopaedics.

Stainless steel is a steel that has a chromium content of between 11% and 30%. The higher amount of chromium gives the steel a relative resistance to many corrosive fluids. The most corrosion-resistant of these stainless steels are those such as 316 low carbon steel. Stainless steel prostheses, usually in the form of wire prostheses, are widely used in middle ear surgery and have proved reliable, particularly when integrated into a mobile ear chain (Figure 4.1). Stainless steel plates have been used for maxillofacial reconstruction and mandibular reconstruction.

Titanium alloys have a reasonable level of corrosion resistance, but often it can be found that the tissue surrounding the implant is dark, indicating an initial loss of titanium to the tissues. Titanium wires are sometimes used in middle ear surgery.

Metal implants if placed against a mobile tympanic membrane will be extruded.

2. Polymers

The first use of a polymer in reconstructive middle ear surgery was in 1952 by Wullstein. He implanted a columella of palavit which gave initially very good hearing results, but in time the implant extruded. Many polymers were subsequently used for different types of columellar reconstruction, but by the end of the 1960s these were largely abandoned as a result of the high extrusion rate.

Many classes of polymers are inappropriate for reconstructive surgery. In otolaryngology the principal generic classes of interest are:

- low density polyethylene (LDPE or LDP);
- high density polyethylene (HDPE or HDP);
- polytetra-fluoroethylene (PTFE, also called Teflon);
- polydimethyl-xylothene (Silastic).

Some polymers also consist of more than one chemical entity. Foreign body reactions occur even to the most tolerant of polymers. A series of toxicity tests are required prior to the introduction of any new polymer. These tests will also assess the tissue reaction to a new material. Long-term animal and clinical studies are required before accepting a new polymer material.

The concept of porous implant materials was developed from the early 1970s. The hope was that these materials would allow ingrowth of fibrous tissue and become integrated into the body. Two porous alloplasts (Proplast and Plastipore) have been promoted in otolaryngology. Proplast is a composite of polytetrafluoroethylene and carbon. Plastipore is a trade name for porous polyethylene polymer.

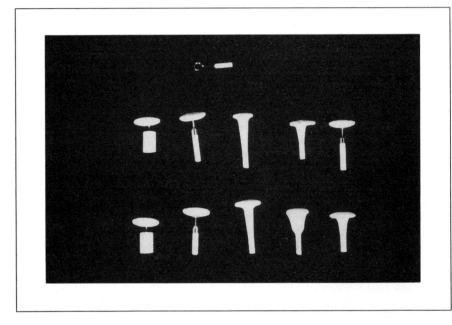

Figure 4.1   This shows a stapedectomy piston at the top of the illustration. These pistons can be constructed with stainless steel, Teflon or an amalgamation of the two substances. The variability of partial and total ossicular replacement prostheses made of hydroxyl apatite are shown in the lower half of the photograph

These porous materials have been designed into total ossicular replacement prosthesis (Torps) and partial ossicular replacement prosthesis (Porps). These have been widely used as columella and middle ear reconstruction devices. On their own these plastipores tend to extrude, but the current belief is that the placement of cartilage between the tympanic membrane and the prosthesis will reduce the rate of extrusion.

Porous materials have been used as implants in maxillofacial surgery. Silastic is often used in otolaryngology within the middle ear as a plastic sheeting. Teflon has been used in the middle ear and can also be used in the head and neck for stenting the larynx and the trachea.

3. Ceramics

Some ceramics are bioinert (most oxide ceramics or a different modification of carbon) while some are bioactive materials (glass ceramics and calcium phosphate ceramics) (Figure 4.1).

- The Al_2O_3 ceramic is a *bioinert* ceramic which is used in otolaryngology. This is a polycrystalline material derived from corundum crystals. This material is very strong and hard. Naturally, because this is a bioinert ceramic, tissue integration is less than with other implant materials, although a fibrous capsule does form. A prosthesis of corundum crystals is difficult to shape, but there has been some clinical success with columellar prostheses. This form of biomaterial behaves well in the middle ear and other applications within maxillofacial surgery may be developed.
- Glass ceramics (*bioactive*) were designed to achieve a direct chemical bond between the implant and living tissues. There are different compositions of surface active glasses (Ceravital, Bioglass and Macor). The reactivity of such ceramics to the body depends on the ion exchange at the surface of the implant material. (The surface of a glass ceramic is coated with an amorphous gel layer which contains silicone dioxide, calcium oxide and phosphorous oxide.) This amorphous gel layer is lysed after implantation as the osteoblasts lay down and embed collagenous fibres. Calcium phosphate precipitates as apatite on the surface and fixes the collagenous fibres on the surface of the implant and thereby prevents further corrosion. All glass ceramics degrade to some extent.

  Glass ceramics are used mainly for middle ear reconstruction in the form of columellar prostheses, but this form of material can be difficult to shape during surgery.
- Calcium phosphate ceramics resemble bone. The problem is that this biomaterial often disappears faster than new bone can fill the empty spaces. In otolaryngology different calcium phosphates of the bone matrix have been studied, in particular B-whitlockite $(Ca_3(PO_4)_2)$ and hydroxylapatite $(Ca_{10}(PO_4)_6(OH)_2)$. Hydroxylapatite is present in the bony tissue, while B-whitlockite is present in the body only in a soluble form. These substances, by means of sintering techniques, can be produced into a ceramic. These calcium phosphate ceramics are very *biocompatible*.

Tricalcium phosphates such as B-whitlockite behave in a similar manner to calcium phosphate in living tissues. The control of degradation and remodelling of these implants is less than with hydroxylapatite. In some instances impurities are present within the ceramic and trace elements of the implant may be found in macrophages around the implant. Tricalcium phosphates (B-whitlockite) have been used for obliteration of mastoid cavities.

Hydroxylapatite has been extensively studied and has a proven track record as a bioactive material which achieves integration with bony tissue without encapsulation. There is contolled remodelling when a porous material is used. These calcium phosphate ceramics can be designed in porous as well as in dense forms. Remodelling of the porous forms continues in the presence of infection. A direct bond and then integration occurs between this material and the surrounding tissue.

Biologically B-whitlockite and hydroxylapatite behave in a similar manner, although the hydroxylapatite is usually less biodegradable. The calcium phosphate materials are resorbed and remodelled in much the same way as a living bone tissue matrix. This resorption and remodelling by macrophages is not only dependent on the surface area of the implant but also on the crystallography and precise chemical design of the ceramic.

The disadvantage of calcium phosphate ceramics is their brittleness. These ceramics have extensive uses within middle ear surgery, both for reconstructive columellar materials and also for reconstruction of the posterior canal wall in mastoid surgery. Currently extensive developments in the fields of nasal and maxillofacial surgery are ongoing.

TISSUE ADHESIVES AND GLUES

An ideal tissue adhesive should have a number of qualities:

1. Ability to spread readily on tissue.
2. Wetability.
3. Minimum heat production.
4. Reasonable polymerization time.
5. Ease of application.
6. A strong and flexible bond.
7. Adequate biodegradability.
8. Minimal histotoxicity.
9. Absent carcinogenesis.
10. Compatibility with wound healing.

There are two principal adhesives available: cyanoacrylate monomers and fibrin glue.

The first generation of cyanoacrylate monomers was abandoned clinically as a result of foreign body histotoxic reaction. Currently N-butyl-2-cyanoacrylate (a long chain monomer) is the only cyanoacrylate tissue adhesive in use today. Its trade name is Histoacryl. This glue has been useful in skin closure in the head and neck with minimal histotoxicity. A spot weld technique gives good skin apposition.

This non-biological glue has also been used in tympanoplastic, dural, vascular repair and for the treatment of corneal ulceration. It may have use in the closure of laryngeal fractures.

Fibrin glue derives from a modification of the coagulation cascade deriving its adhesive properties from the conversion of highly concentrated fibrinogen to fibrin at the gluing site. Two forms of this glue exist:

1. A commercially produced product derived from blood bank factors. This substance carries a small risk of transmission of viral disease such as hepatitis and AIDS.
2. An autologous fibrin tissue adhesive which can be made from each patient's own blood. This glue requires organization for it to be prepared prior to surgery.

Fibrin glue has a number of potential uses in otolaryngology, head and neck surgery, which include:

- Glue ossicular prosthesis and tympanoplastic techniques.
- Posterior canal wall reconstruction.
- Mastoid cavity obliteration.
- Closure of CSF leaks.
- Skin graft placement.
- Closure of 'wound spaces' following neck surgery.

CONCLUSIONS

In conclusion, when considering the choice of implant material one should attempt to choose something which will closely resemble the tissue it is designed to replace, in terms of size, shape and consistency. The material should be structured in such a way that neither infection nor healing reaction will alter its characteristics, and as the implant becomes established it will assume the characteristics of the tissue which it replaces or augments, thereby guaranteeing its permanent place in the body.

Chapter 5

Procedures in the accident and emergency department

INTRODUCTION

Most procedures carried out in the accident department are performed with local or no anaesthesia. Although no formal consent form is used, in most departments the patient implies consent by his or her actions. Nevertheless, it is important to give an adequate explanation of the procedure and any risks that the patient might consider relevant.

NASAL CAUTERY

Indications

Minor epistaxis from prominent vessels on the nasal septum or other points clearly visible on anterior rhinoscopy.

Risks

1. Mucosal ulceration with crusting.
2. Septal performation.
3. Caustic burns of the upper lip, especially when trichloroacetic acid is used; may cause permanent scars.

Preparation

The nose is prepared with a topical anaesthetic and vasoconstrictor solution. Good illumination and running suction are essential.

Method

1. A large aural speculum is inserted into the nares.

2. It is advisable not to burn the vessel directly but to cauterize immediately on either side. This can help to prevent the vessel bursting and starting to bleed. Cautery can be effected with a hot wire or fused silver nitrate on the end of a wire or stick. It is advisable not to cauterize both sides of the septum at corresponding points to prevent a perforation.
3. Excessive use of cautery should be avoided. If necessary the procedure should be repeated several weeks later.

Post-operative care

The patient is advised not to interfere with the nose for several days, but to let any scabs separate naturally. Antiseptic ointment can be of use to reduce vestibular irritation.

ANTERIOR NASAL PACKING

Indications

Active epistaxis.

Risks

1. Trauma to the nasal mucosa, which may lead to intra-nasal adhesions.
2. Sinus infection.
3. Nasal obstruction may lead to hypoxia in a patient with chronic chest disease.
4. Inhalation of the pack.
5. Swallowing the pack. If the pack is soaked in bismuth iodoform paraffin paste this may lead to iodoform toxicity.
6. Otitis media.
7. Rarely trauma to the anterior cranial fossa may occur with the possible risk of CSF leak.
8. Fracture of the middle or inferior turbinate may occur.

Preparation

The nose is prepared with local anaesthetic and vasoconstrictor solution. In patients bleeding torrentially this may be impossible. Good illumination and running suction are essential.

Method

Ribbon gauze soaked in antiseptic and lubricated with liquid paraffin is still the most effective material for controlling epistaxis. Nasal tampons or balloons can be used; they are certainly easier to insert. Usually between 0.6 and 1.2 m of 2.5 cm tape is required.

The gauze is inserted using Tilley's nasal dressing forceps. The pack is pushed to the back of the nose and layers of tape built up until the nasal cavity is packed. The second side is packed. The layering of the pack is shown in Figure 5.1. The two halves of the pack should be joined across the columella. Should the pack be swallowed or inhaled this gives a piece of pack to catch hold of to pull it out. On inserting the pack the forceps tip should always be directed downwards and backwards.

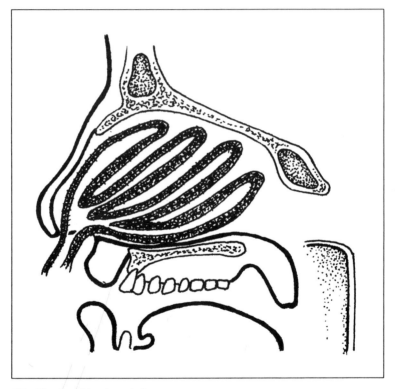

Figure 5.1   Nasal packing (anterior)

Post-operative care

1. If it is expected that the pack may be kept in place for more than 48 hours a prophylactic antibiotic should be prescribed.
2. Daily monitoring of haemoglobin is required, even when a pack is in place, until the bleeding and any subsequent haemodilution has stabilized.

POSTERIOR NASAL PACKING

Indications

Epistaxis that is not controlled by anterior nasal packing.

Risks

1. 1–7 listed under anterior nasal packing.
2. Oedema of the palate and uvula.
3. Ulceration of the skin of the columella.

Preparation

If possible this procedure should be carried out under general anaesthesia, especially in children. However, in cases of severe haemorrhage it may be performed under topical anaesthesia. Running suction should be available.

Method

1. The pack is prepared from a gauze roll with three tapes stitched to it. The roll is impregnated with an antiseptic.
2. A soft rubber catheter is passed through each side of the nose and led out of the mouth. A tape is tied to each catheter and the knot trimmed. The patient is asked to bite on a short dental post or on a gauze roll placed between the back teeth. In a smooth movement the catheters and attached tapes are pulled back through the nose. At the same time a finger is inserted into the patient's mouth and the pack tucked into the postnasal space behind the palate. The third tape is led out of the mouth and taped to the cheek. A 1 cm piece of rubber catheter is threaded over one of the nasal tapes. The two nasal tapes are tied together and the little piece of rubber catheter slid over the knot to prevent pressure ulceration of the columella. This is shown in Figure 5.2.
3. An anterior nasal pack is inserted.
4. Prophylactic antibiotics are prescribed.

Post-operative care

A patient is uncomfortable with a post-nasal pack in place. Sedative drugs may compound 'latent' hypoxia and therefore should be used sparingly. The patient should be admitted to hospital for close observation and prescribed analgesia.

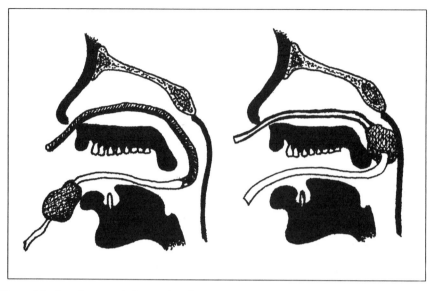

Figure 5.2   Inserting a posterior nasal pack

EAR SYRINGING

Indications

1. Total obstruction of the external auditory canal by ear wax.
2. Removal of an insect that has been killed by instillation of alcohol.
3. Ear wax thought to be causing discomfort.
4. Hearing loss due to ear wax (total occlusion or splintage of the tympanic membrane).
5. To facilitate examination of an obscured tympanic membrane.
6. Ear wax associated with tinnitus.
7. To clear debris in cases of otitis externa. The canal must be subsequently dried.

Contra-indications

1. Non-occlusive ear wax.
2. Previous ear surgery.
3. An only hearing ear.
4. Young children.
5. History of otitis externa following previous syringing.
6. History of chronic otitis media.
7. History of perforation of the tympanic membrane.

Risks

1. Failure to remove the ear wax.
2. The development of otitis externa.
3. Perforation of the tympanic membrane.
4. Trauma to the external auditory canal.
5. Pain.
6. Vertigo.
7. Ossicular damage.
8. Damage to the inner ear (rare).

Preparation

A wax solvent may be used for several days. Oily drops or 5% sodium bicarbonate ear drops are preferable to many proprietary brands. It is important to realize that ear syringing is one of the commonest sources of medical negligence litigation in otolaryngology. If it is delegated to non-medical staff it is essential that they are adequately trained.

Method

1. Water at 37°C should be used. The syringe should be checked. The plunger should run smoothly and the nozzle should be secure.
2. The water jet is directed towards the posterosuperior part of the ear canal (Figure 5.3) and not aimed at the tympanic membrane. Excessive pressure should be avoided. A commercial pulsed water jet may be used.

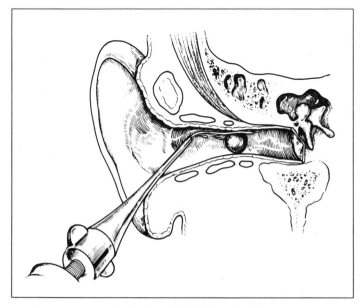

Figure 5.3 Technique for ear syringing (from RSE, by permission)

Post-operative care

The ear canal should be gently dried with cotton wool at the end of the procedure.

AURAL PACKING AND TOILET

Indications

1. Therapy for otitis externa.
2. Following major ear surgery.
3. Following aural polypectomy.

Risks

Complications are rare.

1. Trauma to the external canal.
2. Pain.
3. Trauma to the tympanic membrane, ossicles and inner ear are extremely rare.

Preparation

Anaesthesia is not usually necessary. Good vision is essential and an operating microscope is often required.

Method

1. It is essential that the patients are adequately instructed so that they do not move during the procedure.
2. Suction is used to clean the canal and facilitate examination.
3. Any dressing should be well lubricated prior to insertion.

REMOVAL OF AN AURAL FOREIGN BODY

Indications

1. Aural foreign body.

Risks

1. Trauma to the external auditory canal, tympanic membrane and ossicles.
2. Otitis externa.

Preparation

In young children and the uncooperative adult this procedure should be performed under general anaesthesia.

Method

1. Solid foreign bodies can be removed by passing a blunt hook over the top of the body and pulling it back.
2. Vegetable material can be syringed out, but if this fails suction and cupped forceps can be used.
3. Smooth ferrous metal foreign bodies or welding slag can be removed by positioning an electromagnet at the external auditory meatus. This may not always work in practice!

REMOVAL OF A NASAL FOREIGN BODY

Indications

1. A nasal foreign body.
2. 'Hearing aid' type button batteries must be removed urgently as they can cause severe tissue necrosis.

Risks

1. Trauma to the nasal mucosa. Damage rarely can occur to the turbinates or to the skull base.
2. Inhalation or ingestion of the foreign body.

Preparation

In young children and the uncooperative adult this procedure should be performed under general anaesthesia.

Method

1. A blunt hook is passed over the top of the foreign body and withdrawn.

2. Forceps are used to grasp the foreign body.
3. A suction catheter may aspirate gelatinous foreign bodies.

INCISION AND DRAINAGE OF A PERITONSILLAR ABSCESS (QUINSY)

Indications

A peritonsillar abscess.

Risks

1. An incorrect diagnosis can cause the most serious problems. A peritonsillar abscess may be mistaken for a parapharyngeal space tumour or an aneurysm.
2. Perforation of the palate.
3. Failure to penetrate the abscess.

Preparation

The patient is sat in a chair leaning slightly forwards. Good illumination from a headlight and running suction should be available. Injudicious use of topical anaesthetic agents may anaesthetize the larynx with a consequent risk of aspiration.

To 'guard' the blade of a scalpel, tape is wrapped around the blade, leaving the terminal 1 cm uncovered. This technique prevents accidental over-penetration of the scalpel blade.

Method

1. A guarded scalpel or a quinsy forceps may be used to lance the quinsy. The instrument is inserted over the maximum point of swelling or at a point two-thirds along an imaginary line drawn between the base of the uvula and the last molar. This is shown in Figure 5.4. The abscess may be opened with artery forceps once it is penetrated. Bacteriology sample should be taken.
2. The patient is encouraged to spit out any pus.

Post-operative care

1. The patient is admitted to hospital and commenced on penicillin (erythromycin is useful in cases of penicillin allergy).

2. The patient should be observed in hospital for spread of infection to the soft tissues of the neck until they begin to recover.
3. Traditionally it is usual to recommend tonsillectomy once the infection has settled. Some surgeons would observe the patient if a single peritonsillar abscess was the only evidence of chronic tonsillar infection.

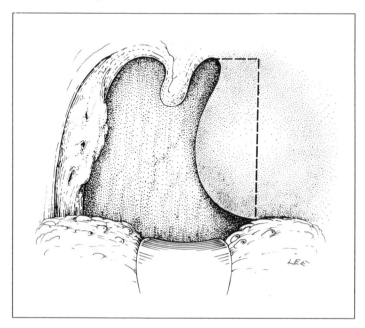

Figure 5.4 Site of incision for quinsy (from RSN, by permission)

MAXILLARY ANTRAL LAVAGE

Indications

1. Acute sinusitis that has failed to resolve.
2. Empyema of the maxillary sinus.
3. Chronic sinusitis. There is debate as to the efficacy of antral washout in this situation.

Contra-indications

1. Hypoplastic maxillary antrum with thick walls.

Risks

1. Nasal haemorrhage.

2. Penetration of the soft tissues of the cheek.
3. Penetration of the orbit.
4. Failure to puncture the antrum.

Preparation

The nose is prepared with topical anaesthetic and vasoconstrictive agents. Good illumination and running suction should be available. In cases of acute sinusitis the procedure is preferably performed under general anaesthesia.

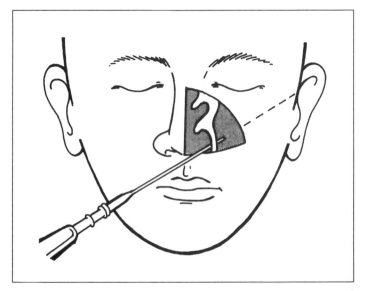

Figure 5.5   Insertion of a trocar and canula for antral lavage (from RSN, by permission)

Method

1. The point of the trocar is inserted *high* under the inferior turbinate and positioned approximately 1 cm behind the anterior end where the bone is thinnest (Figure 5.5). The trocar is directed towards the tragus on that side. The antrum is penetrated using steady pressure. An extended finger acts as a guard to prevent inserting the trocar too far.
2. The cannula can be advanced to palpate gently the walls of the maxillary antrum and identify polypoid tissue.
3. A 20 ml syringe half filled with normal saline is attached to the cannula. The barrel of the syringe is withdrawn and air should then enter the syringe if the cannula is in the correct position. If nothing is withdrawn this may be because the natural ostium is closed. In this situation a second cannula is inserted alongside the first. Once it has been confirmed that the cannula is in place, a small amount of lavage solution is injected whilst the thumb of the other hand rests on the closed eye, feeling for any proptosis. Provided no pain is experienced and no swelling observed, lavage may commence.

4. Under local anaesthesia the patient is sat leaning forward. The patient is given a bowl to hold. The cannula is connected to a Higginson's syringe. The lavage is commenced and the fluid is allowed to run out of the mouth and nose to be caught in the bowl. Under general anaesthesia the patient is not leant forward but the lavage fluid is aspirated from the nose and mouth using a sucker. A washout sample is sent for bacteriological examination.

REDUCING A NASAL FRACTURE

Indications

1. Nasal fracture with deviation of the nasal bones. Manipulations should ideally be performed within 2 weeks of the injury, but may be considered up to 6 weeks from the initial trauma.

Risks

1. Haemorrhage.
2. Aspiration of blood in cases of severe haemorrhage.
3. Failure to reduce the fracture.
4. Trauma to the skin from external dressings.
5. Risks associated with nasal packing.
6. Conjunctivitis from plaster dust.
7. Septal haematoma or abscess. These complications may lead to a saddle deformity of the nasal bridge.
8. Nasal infection.
9. Intra-nasal adhesions. These are rare. They may be divided and silastic splints inserted for 7 days to prevent recurrence.

Preparation

1. General peroral endotracheal anaesthesia with a throat pack inserted is commonly used for this procedure, although in some stoical adults local anaesthesia may be applied.
2. The nasal cavity should be prepared with topical anaesthetic and vasoconstrictor spray.
3. A local regional anaesthetic block can be effected. The infratrochlear, external nasal, medial branches of the infraorbital and nasal branches of the greater palatine nerves are blocked.
4. Good illumination and running suction should be available.

Method

1. The nose is carefully inspected to assess the injury. Walsham's forceps are used to disimpact the nasal bones. Initially the processes are displaced laterally and the deformity increased.

2. By using Walsham's forceps and forward traction the nasal bones are disimpacted.
3. The septum may be relocated with Asch's forceps. It is not uncommon to find this manoeuvre difficult.
4. The fingers are used to mould the nasal skeleton back to shape.
5. When the septum does not reduce to a satisfactory position an open reduction may be necessary using septoplasty techniques.
6. External lacerations are stitched after thorough cleansing.
7. If the reshaped nose is 'unstable' then an external splint is applied.
8. External fixation is effected with tape to the skin. The strips should overlap by 50%. Plaster of Paris strips may be applied. Great care should be taken to avoid getting plaster dust in the eyes. A 'stent' material may be used which may be shaped after softening in hot water. The cast is attached by adhesive tape.
9. In depressed fractures where there is severe comminution of the fragments, lead plates may be attached externally using steel sutures, which are passed with a Keith needle. This technique allows lateral pressure to be applied and is illustrated in Figure 5.6.
10. Fractures may also be reduced using an open technique. Long-standing deformities require a septorhinoplasty.

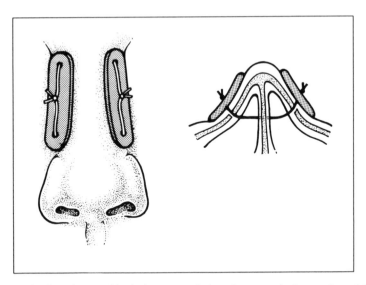

Figure 5.6 Fixation of external lead plates to apply lateral pressure in depressed nasal fractures (from RSN, by permission)

Post-operative care

1. Analgesia.
2. Ice packs may reduce periorbital haematomas.
3. Any nasal packs should be removed within 2 days. Packs should be avoided when there is CSF rhinorrhoea.

4. Plaster splints are removed after 10–14 days.
5. Lateral lead splints are removed after 21 days unless sepsis intervenes.
6. Prophylactic antibiotics are required when there is a CSF leak or an open fracture.

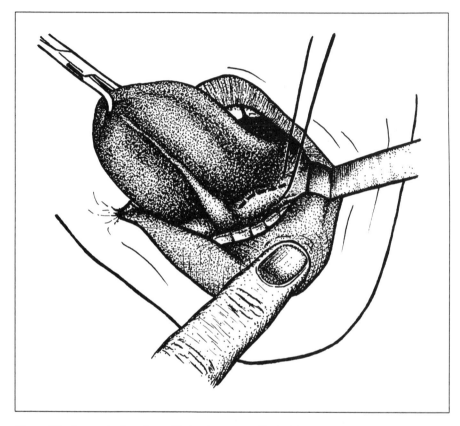

Figure 5.7 Removal of a submandibular duct stone. The incision line is shown over the stone

REMOVAL OF A SUBMANDIBULAR DUCT STONE

Indications

1. Stone in the submandibular duct. Stones in the gland are best dealt with by gland excision.

Risks

1. Damage to the lingual nerve.
2. Duct stenosis.

Preparation

Lingual nerve block or general anaesthesia. Good illumination and running suction should be available.

Method

1. The mouth is propped open. The tongue is retracted to the opposite side. A traction suture may be used for this. The stone is palpated. A suture is passed deep to the duct proximal to the stone. A single throw is tied to prevent the stone moving. This is shown in Figure 5.7.
2. The duct is slit open longitudinally to reveal the stone, which is removed.
3. The duct is irrigated to wash out any fragments. The duct is not closed.
4. Fine non-absorbable sutures may be used to stitch the incision 'open'. This prevents subsequent stenosis.

Post-operative care

1. Antiseptic or salt mouth washes.
2. Massage of the gland to promote saliva flow.
3. Antibiotics are prescribed if the gland is infected.

Chapter 6

Procedures most common in children

TONSILLECTOMY

Indications

1. Repeated attacks of tonsillitis. It is important to establish that the patient has been having tonsillitis rather than viral pharyngitis. Many surgeons consider that four attacks per year for two years, or six attacks in any one year, are reasonable guidelines as a definition of 'repeated tonsillitis'. However, severity of attacks, social and educational effects, and the parents' or child's wishes should be taken into consideration. It is important to remember that most young children lose time from school due to tonsillitis. This problem often resolves without surgery. Repeated tonsillar infections often occur in the first year at school and it is wise to avoid any decision about tonsillectomy at this time.
2. Quinsy. One peritonsillar abscess may be considered an adequate reason to offer tonsillectomy. Many surgeons would review a patient after 6 months if one episode of peritonsillar abscess was the sole evidence of tonsillar disease. A patient with a quinsy that fails to resolve after drainage and adequate antibiotic therapy has a very strong case for tonsillectomy.
3. Biopsy for suspected malignancy.
4. As part of the surgical approach to structures deep to the tonsil bed such as the glossopharyngeal nerve or styloid process.
5. Tonsillitis that frequently leads to acute otitis media or exacerbation or tubotympanic disease of the middle ear cleft.
6. Obstructive sleep apnoea. In adults this may be combined with a uvulopalatoplasty where the obstruction is due to oro- and nasopharyngeal factors.

Contra-indications

1. Patients with a suspected bleeding disorder should be thoroughly investigated. Any deficit should be corrected in consultation with a haematologist prior to surgery.
2. Patients with a religious objection to blood transfusion should be carefully

counselled. Tonsillectomy is rarely performed for life-threatening reasons, but it has life-threatening complications.

3. Children incubating an infectious disease or with a concurrent upper respiratory tract infection.
4. Children who have not been immunized against polio and there is a concurrent polio epidemic.

Risks

1. Haemorrhage (primary and secondary).
2. Dental damage, diathermy burns.
3. Cervical spine damage, particularly in Down's syndrome.
4. Palatal scarring which may rarely lead to rhinolalia aperta or nasal regurgitation.
5. Parapharyngeal abscess.

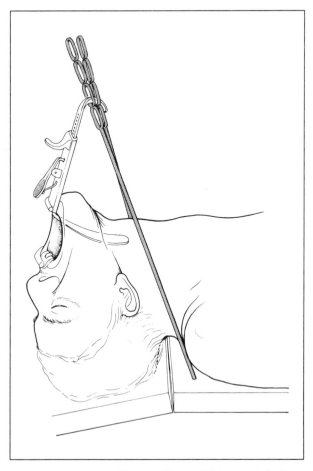

Figure 6.1   Patient positioned for tonsillectomy (from RSN, by permission)

Preparation

1. General anaesthesia delivered through peroral intubation in children. Nasal intubation can be used in adults. A headlight should be used for illumination and running suction should be available. The operation can be performed under local anaesthesia in rare cases.
2. The patient is supine with the neck extended by a sand bag placed under the shoulders. A Boyle–Davis gag is inserted and opened with the tongue plate in the mid line. The gag can be suspended on a Draffin bipod or a cord suspended from the operating room ceiling. This position is shown in Figure 6.1.
3. The tonsillar fossae can be infiltrated with 1–2% lignocaine with 1:200 000 adrenaline to facilitate dissection and reduce haemorrhage. This is not a commonly used technique.

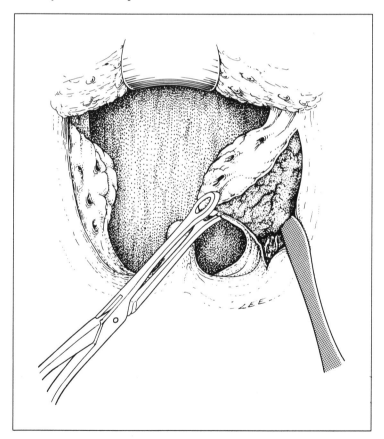

Figure 6.2 Mobilization of the tonsil (from RSN, by permission)

Method

1. The tonsil is grasped and pulled medially. An incision is made on the medial edge of the anterior faucial pillar to reveal the tonsil capsule.

2. Blunt dissection opens the capsular plane. Using both blunt and sharp dissection, the upper pole is freed. The tonsil is separated from its bed from superior to inferior whilst traction is maintained (Figure 6.2).
3. The fibrous lower pole is freed by sharp dissection. The tonsil is finally detached by snare (Figure 6.3).
4. Haemorrhage is controlled. Minor ooze stops due to vessel contraction. Diathermy or ligatures are used on persistent bleeding vessels. Once bleeding has been stopped the pressure from the gag on the base of the tongue is released to see if any further bleeding starts.

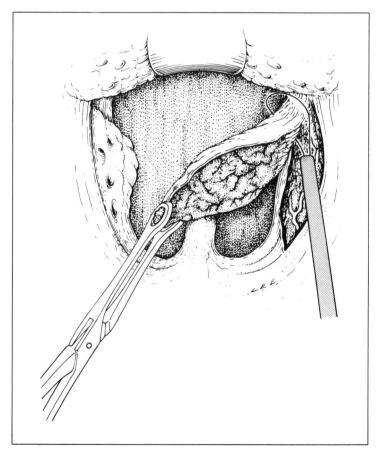

Figure 6.3 Using the snare to detach the tonsil (from RSN, by permission)

Post-operative care

1. The patient is recovered on his or her side in a slight head-down position and supervised closely until full consciousness is reached.

2. Adequate analgesia, initially with a narcotic and subsequently with minor painkillers such as ibuprofen or paracetamol, is provided.
3. Primary haemorrhage is dealt with in the operating room. In the early stages the only sign of bleeding in the sleeping child can be repeated swallowing. Occasionally the problem may present with haematemesis.
4. The patient should be encouraged to eat and drink in order to keep the tonsillar beds clean and reduce the risk of infection.

Treatment of post-tonsillectomy haemorrhage

1. Primary haemorrhage is usually brisk and occurs at the time of surgery or in the immediate post-operative period. In this case the patient should be returned to the operating room promptly after an intravenous infusion has been inserted and resuscitation commenced. The patient should be stabilized by intravenous infusion with a plasma expander whilst blood is being cross-matched. Once stable, an experienced surgeon and anaesthetist control the bleeding in the operating room. Ligatures, diathermy or undersewing may be required. Occasionally the anterior and posterior pillars have to be sewn over a swab for 24 hours, but this should only be used as a last resort because of the potential risk of inhalation or swallowing the swab.
2. Secondary haemorrhage is usually minor. Any clot should be removed. Weak hydrogen peroxide (1–2 volume) gargles can be used for that purpose. Care should be taken over the use of hydrogen peroxide gargles in children. The patient is commenced on antibiotics (usually penicillin). Occasionally secondary bleeding can be severe.

Management of complications

1. A dental opinion should be sought if dentition is damaged.
2. Parapharyngeal abscess should be drained via an external neck incision and the patient commenced on intravenous antibiotics.

ADENOIDECTOMY

Indications

1. Established otitis media with effusion in the presence of a reduced nasal airway. Most authorities recommend that the effusion is affecting both ears and has been present for at least 3 months. A significant hearing loss should also be present.
2. Repeated attacks of acute otitis media associated with nasal obstruction due to enlarged adenoids.
3. Severe nasal obstruction due to enlarged adenoids. This should be differentiated from nasal obstruction due to engorged turbinates. It should also be considered that most children will 'grow out' of this condition.
4. Biopsy in cases of suspected neoplasia of the lymphatic system.

Risks

1.   As for tonsillectomy, but palatal scarring is rare.
2.   Rhinolalia aperta. To minimize this risk adenoidectomy should not be performed in the presence of cleft palate. Adenoidectomy should be very carefully considered when a submucosal cleft palate is present.

Preparation

General anaesthesia delivered through peroral intubation. The patient is positioned as for a tonsillectomy.

Method

1.   The adenoid is carefully palpated to feel for any pulsation or unusual texture that might indicate that the tissue in the post-nasal space was neoplastic.
2.   An adenoid curette is passed over the adenoid and embedded into the tissue (Figure 6.4). The adenoid is then removed by sweeping the curette into the oropharynx. Any adenoid tags are felt for and removed with the curette. Care should be taken that the area of the Eustachian tube orifices is not traumatized lest scar tissue might obstruct the tubes.
3.   A swab with a 'tail' is inserted into the post-nasal space and left for a few minutes.
4.   The swab is removed. Bleeding usually stops spontaneously. If bleeding persists this is usually from retained tags, which should be removed. If bleeding still persists despite the patience of the surgeon then the adenoid bed should be inspected with the aid of a mirror. Using a palate retractor and angled diathermy forceps, any bleeding vessel can usually be diathermized. Rarely bleeding may still persist and if this is the case a post-nasal pack should be inserted.
5.   It is useful to pass a soft catheter through the nose if there is any doubt as to nasal patency. Occasionally a unilateral choanal atresia can be found this way.

Post-operative care

The same as for tonsillectomy.

Management of complications

1.   Haemorrhage is managed, in general, the same way as for a post-tonsillectomy haemorrhage. A post-nasal pack may be required.
2.   Infective complications are managed the same way as for tonsillectomy.

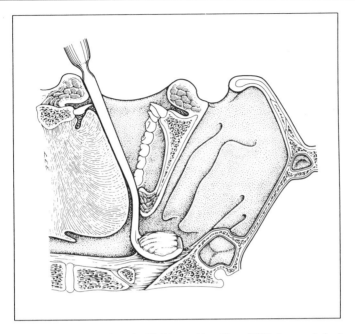

Figure 6.4 The adenoid curette is embedded in position (from RSN, by permission)

MYRINGOTOMY AND VENTILATION TUBE INSERTION

Indications for myringotomy alone

1. Acute otitis media (circumferential incision).
2. Acute barotraumatic otitis media.
3. To facilitate a transtympanic biopsy.

Indications for myringotomy with ventilation tube insertion

4. Established otitis media with effusion.
5. Repeated episodes of barotraumatic otitis media.
6. To facilitate the injection of drugs into the middle ear in the treatment of Meniere's disease.
7. To relieve the sensation of 'fullness' that can occur in Meniere's disease.

Risks

Significant complications are rare.

1. Damage can occur to the ossicular chain, a high jugular bulb or a dehiscent facial nerve.

2.   A ventilation tube may be dropped through the myringotomy and 'lost' in the middle ear.
3.   The ear may continuously discharge via the tube if there is a chronic cholesterol granuloma involving the mastoid or middle ear.
4.   Tympanosclerosis affecting the tympanic membrane is a very common occurrence which increases with time even after the ventilation tube has been extruded. This form of tympanosclerosis rarely causes any significant hearing impairment.
5.   Infection. This can be an immediate post-operative or a late complication. Soapy water has a low surface tension and will easily pass through the tube. This is believed to be an aetiological factor in some infections. Many surgeons permit their patients to swim provided that ear protection is worn and that diving and under-water activities are avoided.
6.   Perforation of tympanic membrane. This usually occurs following the extrusion of 'long stay' ventilation tubes such as 'T' tubes.
7.   Obstruction of the ventilation tube by wax or dried effusion.
8.   Profuse haemorrhage can occur in the very rare instance of a patient with an ectopic carotid artery passing through the middle ear.

Preparation

1.   In children a general anaesthetic is required. In co-operative adults local anaesthesia may be used. An operating microscope is required. Running suction should be available.

Method

1.   The surgery is performed permeatally via a speculum. Rarely the external auditory canal can be very narrow (not an uncommon finding in Down's syndrome). In this situation a small endaural incision will improve access.
2.   The ear drum and attic region should be thoroughly inspected.
3.   (Figure 6.5). A radial incision is made with a myringotome in the anterior half of the drum. It is believed that a circumferential incision takes longer to heal than a radial incision and is therefore useful in acute otitis media. The incisions are shown in Figure 6.5. If the access to the anterior half of the drum is restricted then the myringotomy can be made in the posterior inferior quadrant, although care should be taken that the blade does not damage underlying structures. A posterior superior myringotomy should be avoided because of the underlying stapes and incudostapedial joint.
4.   When it is the intention to insert a ventilation tube any obvious fluid in the middle ear should be aspirated lest it dry and obstruct the grommet. In cases where the effusion is very thick and tenacious a few drops of hypertonic urea placed in the ear will facilitate aspiration. Care should be taken not to traumatize the drum.
5.   There are many different designs of ventilation tube. Shepard and Shah tubes stay in place from 6–18 months; Armstrong and Reuter bobbins stay in place 12–48 months; 'T' tubes or Per Lee tubes can stay in place

indefinitely. The manufacturers usually describe a technique for inserting their tube or they have an instrument which facilitates insertion.

6. Once in place the patency of the tube should be verified. If the external auditory canal is bleeding from a minor abrasion the blood may obstruct the tube. A moist piece of ribbon gauze can be inserted into the external canal and removed several hours later to prevent a blood obstructed ventilation tube.

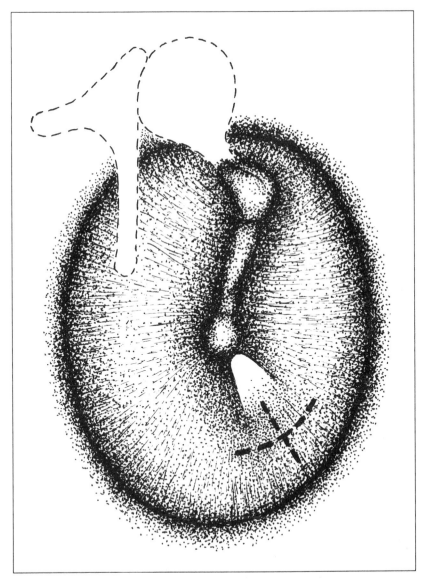

Figure 6.5 The radial incision for grommet insertion and the circumferential incision for acute otitis media

Post-operative care

1. Any dressings are removed after several hours. It is useful to establish that the patient has noticed an improvement in hearing prior to discharge from hospital.
2. Advice is given concerning soapy water and swimming.
3. Antibiotics are prescribed if the middle ear is infected.
4. A pure tone audiogram should be performed at the first hospital visit after surgery to ensure that a sensorineural hearing loss has not been masked by a conductive deafness.

PINNAPLASTY

Indications

1. A protrusion of the external ear. Ridicule may precipitate the desire for surgery. The ideal time for surgical correction is the year before starting school in order to minimize the psychological trauma.

Risks

1. Haematoma which may lead to a 'cauliflower' deformity if not aspirated and treated.
2. Infection. This may lead to perichondritis and subsequent deformity.
3. Failure to correct the deformity.

Preparation

General anaesthesia delivered through an endotracheal tube. In the adult the procedure may be performed under local anaesthesia. The skin is prepared with antiseptic and the patient draped.

Method

1. The pinna is folded back and the created antihelix is marked by piercing the pinna with a dye laden needle.
2. The medial surface of the pinna is infiltrated with a vasoconstrictive solution such as 1:200 000 adrenaline.
3. A dumb bell ellipse of skin is excised from the medial aspect of the pinna.
4. The skin is undermined towards the free edge of the pinna. The cartilage of the pinna is incised along the border of the pinna just immediately proximal to the helix (Figure 6.6,). The skin is elevated from the lateral aspect of the pinna until the dye marks of the new antihelix have been passed by about 2–3 mm.

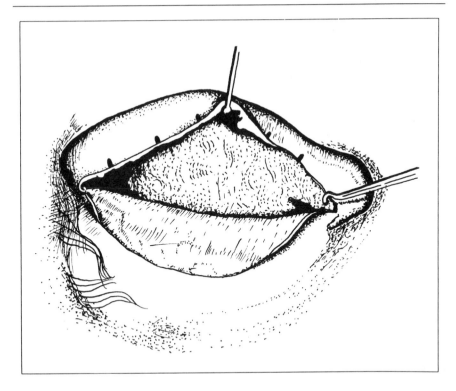

Figure 6.6 Elevation of the postauricular skin from the pinna

5. The perichondrium is scored to break the cartilage spring in such a way as to create a new antihelix. The cartilage may be incised full thickness at the inferior end just above the origin of the ear lobe (Figure 6.7).
6. The skin is replaced. Great attention is paid to haemostasis using bipolar diathermy. The postauricular incision is closed with a subcuticular suture.
7. Antiseptic soaked wool is wrapped around the ears and a gauze and crepe dressing is applied.

This technique is one of many. It requires modification of approach for other deformities such as lop ear. Other techniques have been described which rely on the insertion of permanent sutures (Mustarde). The technique described above gives a reasonable result in most cases, but it is not easy to get excellent results in every case.

Post-operative care

1. The dressings and sutures are removed between 10 and 14 days. Some surgeons prescribe prophylactic flucloxacillin.
2. Severe pain may indicate the presence of an infection. The dressings should be removed and the ears inspected.

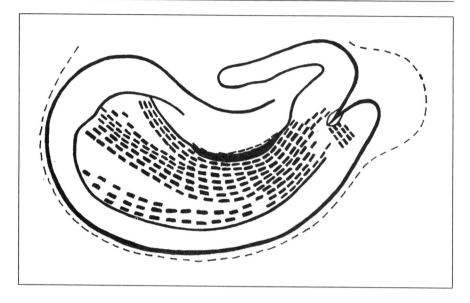

Figure 6.7   Anterior surface of conchal cartilage illustrating lines of scoring

SURGERY FOR CHOANAL ATRESIA

Indications

Unilateral or bilateral choanal atresia.

Introduction

In the newborn, choanal atresia can present as an emergency with apparent total apnoea until the mouth is opened and an airway inserted. In the emergency situation an airway can be taped in place to avoid intubation. Often unilateral choanal atresia is not diagnosed until later in childhood or even adult life.

A simple test for nasal patency is to place a mirror under the nostrils and to observe the misting pattern. Confirmation of the diagnosis can be reached by failure to pass a fine catheter into the nasopharynx. Radiology can help delineate the extent of the atresia and identify whether it is membranous or bony.

Risks

1. The basisphenoid can be penetrated in removing the superior portion of the obstructive plate. A CSF leak can result.
2. Haemorrhage may occur, especially from the sphenopalatine artery.

3. A secondary sinusitis may develop from long-term intra-nasal tubes.
4. Loss of the palatal flap and naso-oral fistula formation following a transpalatal approach.
5. The complications associated with a Caldwell–Luc operation when this approach is used.

Preparation

The child is positioned and prepared as for a tonsillectomy.

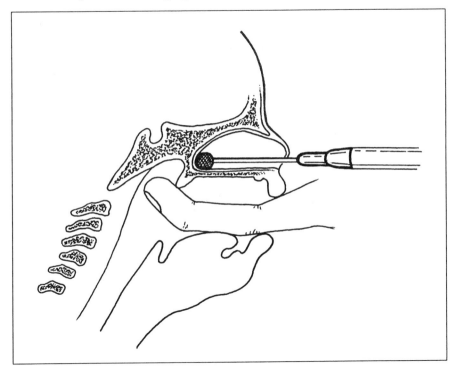

Figure 6.8 Technique for penetration of the choanal septum

Method

1. A finger is placed in the post-nasal space. A sleeved cutting burr loaded in a drill is introduced via the nares and used to perforate the bony obstruction. The finger in the post-nasal space is used to guide the direction of the drill. It is important to keep the drill parallel with the floor of the nose. This is shown in Figure 6.8.
2. A larger diamond burr is used to enlarge the posterior choanae. A mirror or Hopkin's rod telescope can be used to inspect the progress of the surgery. It is important that a portion of the posterior end of the vomer is removed.

3. A length of 12 FG nasogastric tube is cut twice the length of the nasal cavity. At the mid point a 1.5 cm length of half the diameter of the tube is excised (Figure 6.9). The tube is looped around the posterior part of the septum. The tube is retained in position for 6 weeks.

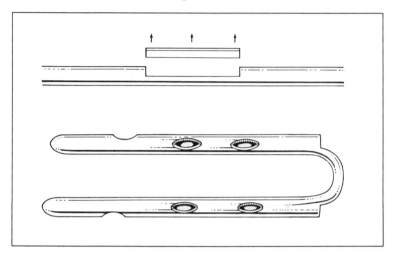

Figure 6.9   Nasal stent tubes for choanal atresia (from RSN, by permission)

Post-operative care

1. The child is recovered on its side.
2. The tubes require regular suction to prevent blockage.

Other techniques

1. In the older child or adult is may be necessary to consider a transpalatal approach, especially if the choanae restenose (Figures 14.5 and 14.6). The U-shaped palatal flap is cut keeping close to the teeth in order to include the arterial supply. The soft palate is detached from the bony palate. A drill is used to remove bone from the free edge of the hard palate. In this way the atretic plate can be exposed with good visibility of the important landmarks. Once the atretic plate has been removed the palatal flap is sutured in place and the tubes are secured in the nose.
2. In an adult with a unilateral atresia the atretic plate can be exposed by first opening the maxillary antrum via a Caldwell–Luc approach. The medial wall of the antrum is then removed and the atretic plate removed.

Chapter 7

Principles of otological surgery

PRE-OPERATIVE PREPARATION

1. Except in the case of an ear with proven total loss of hearing, an audiogram should be performed within 3 months of the operation, or ideally within a week of surgery.
2. Care should be taken that the patient understands the reason for the proposed surgery and the potential for benefit. He or she should be aware of the likely success and risks of the surgery. The important points to cover include:

   - Peri-operative course.
   - Length of absence from school or work.
   - Restrictions on flying, swimming and hair washing.
   - Specific operative risks.

   The surgeon should know his or her own success rate for the surgery involved so a frank discussion can take place. It is important to explain what would be the likely outcome if the patient chose to avoid surgery.
3. The patient should have a bath and hair wash on the day of surgery. The surgeon should give instructions concerning the shaving of hair from around the ear. Shaving is not required for permeatal surgery unless it is envisaged that a temporalis fascia graft will be required. When an endaural approach is proposed then about 3 cm of hair should be shaved from above the ear and 2 cm from in front of the ear. In a post-aural approach for mastoidectomy 5 cm at least should be shaved from behind the ear and 3 cm from above the ear. It is a good guide to consider that the hair should be removed so that there is at least 2 cm of shaved skin around the incision. Consequently when a temporalis muscle flap is envisaged or the surgeon intends to remove an acoustic neuroma as much as half of the head may need to be shaved. Usually the shave can be performed on the ward prior to surgery, but in children or when a large shave is required it can be performed after general anaesthesia has been induced.
4. Consent should be taken for the surgery and anaesthetic. This should be tailored for the individual operation and patient.
5. When the patient goes to the operating room the ward nursing staff should ensure that all records, audiograms and radiographs accompany the patient.

SKIN PREPARATION

1. The skin is usually prepared with an antiseptic solution prior to placement of towels. When there is a perforation of the tympanic membrane it is wise to plug the external auditory canal with a piece of sterile cotton wool prior to cleaning the skin. The skin may be prepared with an aqueous solution or an alcohol-based solution. However, little puddles of alcohol can collect in the pinna and subsequently be ignited by diathermy. The operative field should be carefully dried when alcohol preparation is used.
2. An iodine-containing solution, such as Betadine, can be used. The thick consistency and soap has the added advantage that any loose strands of hair can be kept clear of the operative site. Post-operative scalp itch can be a problem when the combination of Betadine and a head bandage are used. For those allergic to iodine a chlorhexidene solution may be used.
3. Many surgeons prefer to use no skin preparation for permeatal surgery, especially if it is intended to open the inner ear. Some surgeons like to wipe the external auditory canal clean with a damp ball of cotton wool.

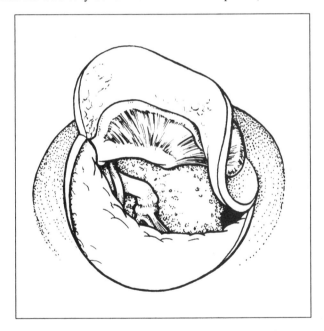

Figure 7.1 The anatomy revealed after elevation of a posterior tympanomeatal flap (from RSE, by permission)

INCISIONS AND APPROACHES

Permeatal approach

This is usually employed for minor surgery on the ear, including:

1. Myringotomy, with or without insertion of ventilation tube.
2. Examination of the ear.
3. Myringoplasty for a central perforation.
4. Stapedectomy.
5. Ossiculoplasty.

The surgeon will require the use of both hands for the more major operation. A speculum is inserted and held in place with a holder that is attached to the operating table.

Posterior tympanomeatal flap

This is a standard approach to the middle ear for tympanoplasty and stapedectomy. It gives excellent access to:

1. Stapes, stapes footplate, incudostapedial joint.
2. The round window area.
3. The promontory.

This is shown in Figure 7.1.

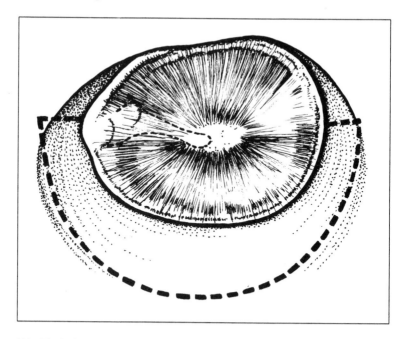

Figure 7.2   The incision for a posterior tympanomeatal flap

Method

1. The external auditory canal should be imagined to be the face of a clock for this description. Twelve o'clock represents the lateral process of the malleus.

2. The skin is infiltrated with local anaesthetic just medial to the cartilaginous bony junction of the external auditory canal in its posterior half.
3. An incision is made from 12 o'clock to 6 o'clock about 4–6 mm lateral to the annulus. A triangular knife or a roller knife can be used for this. A vertical incision is made from 12 o'clock to the annulus. A second incision is made from 6 o'clock to the annulus. The vertical and horizontal incisions should connect (Figure 7. 2).
4. The suction is turned to the lowest pressure. In this way any blood may be aspirated without traumatizing the flap.
5. An elevator is used to raise the flap. A small ball of cotton wool can be used to protect the flap. Any strands of skin or fibrous tissue can be cut with microscissors.
6. Once the annulus is reached a curved needle is used to dislocate the tympanic membrane. This should be performed at the posterior inferior quadrant. Thus the middle ear is entered at the level of the round window.
7. An elevator is inserted and the annulus is dislocated superiorly to reveal the incudostapedial joint. The flap is turned forward; it can be protected by a cotton wool ball from damage during surgery. Sometimes it is necessary to dissect the chorda tympani nerve free from the tympanic membrane with the use of a curved needle before the ear drum will 'turn' easily forwards.
8. If there is a perforation in the membrane then the edges should be excised or freshened with a needle prior to elevating the annulus.

Endaural approach

This approach gives access to the same structures as the permeatal approach, but by widening the external auditory canal, vision and instrument handling are improved.

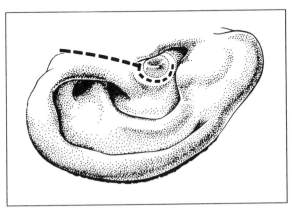

Figure 7.3 The endaural incision (from RSE, by permission)

If the incision is extended superiorly or over the top of the ear the temporalis muscle can be exposed in order that a fascia graft can be taken. This incision is shown in Figures 7.3 and 7.4. Extending the incision superiorly and then posteriorly over the top of the pinna gives access to the outer attic wall, mastoid antrum and mastoid. Thus an atticotomy or atticoantrostomy can be performed, as shown in Figure 7.5. Access is usually inadequate to perform a mastoidectomy in the well pneumatized bone.

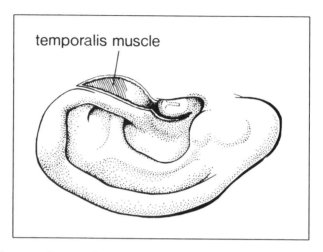

Figure 7.4   Exposure of temporalis muscle via the endaural incision (from RSE, by permission)

Method

1. The skin may be infiltrated with local anaesthetic and vasoconstrictor solution.
2. The incision runs anterior to the root of the helix, then posterior to the tragus at the 12 o'clock position. It can be extended down to the annulus or round the posterior aspect of the meatus from 12 to 6 o'clock.

Post-auricular incision

This curving incision gives access to the entire mastoid bone, the external auditory canal, tympanum, facial nerve and inner ear structures. Consequently it is used for mastoidectomy, myringoplasty, ossiculoplasty, facial nerve exploration from the geniculate ganglion to the stylomastoid foramen, semicircular canal surgery, posterior tympanotomy, saccus endolymphaticus surgery and the translabyrinthine approach to the internal auditory canal.

Method

1. The skin may be infiltrated with local anaesthetic and vasoconstrictive solution.
2. A curving incision commences from just above the pinna round to the mastoid tip (Figure 7.6). This incision is made about a centimetre posterior to the sulcus. This incision is deepened to the plane between the deep fascia

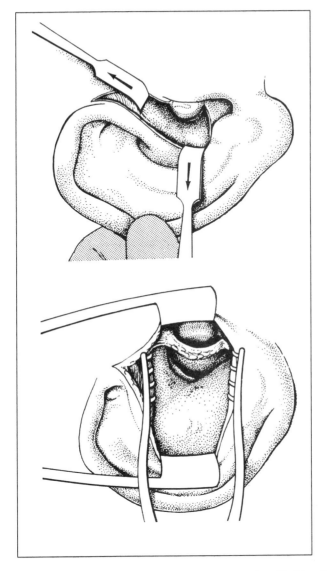

Figure 7.5 Exposure of the mastoid, and outer attic wall, via the endaural incision (from RSE, by permission)

and the temporalis fascia. The anterior flap consisting of the skin and pinna is elevated to reveal the root of the zygoma and the soft tissues of the external auditory canal.

3. If necessary a superior flap can be elevated to reveal the fascia of the temporalis muscle for harvesting of a graft.

4. To reveal the mastoid bone a posterior based periosteal flap is cut (Figure 7.7). The superior incision runs along the edge of the temporalis muscle. The anterior incision runs from the zygomatic root round the bony margin of the external auditory canal. The inferior limb runs backwards over the

mastoid at the point where the sternomastoid muscle is attached. The lines of these incisions are shown in Figure 7.7. A periosteal elevator is then used to reveal the bare bone. The flaps are held back using self-retaining retractors and stay sutures as necessary.

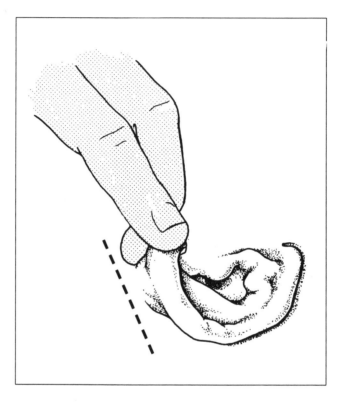

Figure 7.6   Modification of the postaural incision for mastoid surgery in infants (from RSE, by permission)

Extensions of the post-auricular incision

1. The post-auricular incision may be extended down into the neck along the anterior border of the sternomastoid. In this way a large anterior flap can be raised, especially if the external auditory canal is transected. In this way the parotid gland can be revealed and a means of access to the jugular foramen, from below, created.
2. The incision may be extended superiorly in a curve over the surface marking of the anterior attachment of the temporalis muscle. This allows a temporalis muscle flap to be created.

Meatoplasty

The purpose of a meatoplasty is to widen the 'soft tissue' external auditory canal. This is believed to improve ventilation of any mastoid cavity that has been created. There are many different types of meatoplasty that have been described. A Koerner meatoplasty is described here.

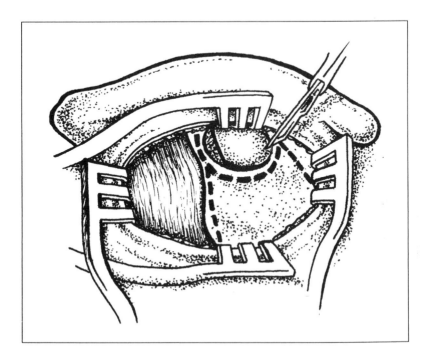

Figure 7.7   This illustrates the periosteal incisions for the posterior based periosteal flap

Method

1. The skin over the conchal cartilage is infiltrated with local anaesthetic and vasoconstrictive solution to ease dissection of the skin from the underlying conchal cartilage.
2. Considering a right ear, two radial incisions are placed from the external meatus at the 8 and 10 o'clock positions.
3. A circumferential incision is made between the radial incision within the ear canal.
4. The skin is elevated from the cartilage and the wax secreting skin at the tip of the flap excised.
5. A 'D' of conchal cartilage is excised (Figure 7.8). The cartilage should be excised from under the superior and inferior flaps; this helps to prevent granulation tissue developing at the incision lines.
6. The soft tissues deep to the cartilage are also excised so that the new meatus opens fully into the cavity. The flap of skin is used partially to line the cavity.

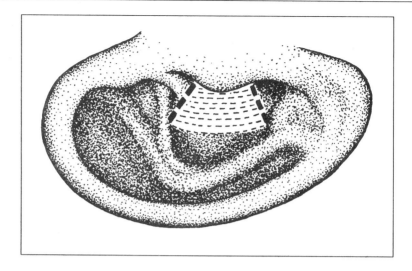

Figure 7.8   Conchal incisions for a Korner meatoplasty. The shaded area is the portion of conchal cartilage to be excised

Harvest of a temporalis fascia graft

Fascia is taken to graft the tympanic membrane or line a mastoid cavity.

Method

1. The muscle is exposed.
2. An incision is made through the fascia to reveal the muscle underneath. An elevator is passed between the muscle and its fascia. It is swept from side to side to divide the tenuous connections between the fascia and muscle. The fascia is excised using scissors or a knife.

Use of the drill

The drill is the surgeon's most important tool in mastoid surgery. Handled correctly it can be used to remove bone to within fractions of a millimetre of important structures. The basic rules of its use are:

1. The largest burr possible should be chosen. Care should be taken to ensure the spinning burr does not come into contact with important structures away from the working area.
2. Adequate irrigation should be used to keep the burr and bone cool. Excessive heating of bone close to the facial nerve may lead to a palsy.
3. The spinning burr should not be advanced blindly into the bone. Bone should be cut by working from deep to superficial or by following the line in which important anatomical structures run.

4. When working close to important structures such as the dura or the facial nerve then a diamond paste burr should be used. When using such a burr copious irrigation should be used. Diamond burrs heat the bone more quickly than steel cutting burrs.
5. The surgeon must have adequate vision of the working area. The use of suction, angled drill hand pieces and appropriate magnification can aid this.
6. When the ossicular chain is intact great care should be taken when working with a drill close to any ossicle. If necessary the incudostapedial joint should be divided. Touching an ossicle with spinning burr can lead to high tone sensory deafness.

Chapter 8

Tympanotomy and tympanoplasty

MYRINGOPLASTY

Introduction

The presence of a perforation of the tympanic membrane in itself is not an indication for surgery. Many patients live with a symptomless perforation without knowing it.

Indications

1. Hearing loss. This is less than 30 dB and is conductive in nature. A greater hearing loss usually indicates an ossicular abnormality.
2. Discharge. This is typically intermittent in nature and often occurs following water contamination of the ear or coincidental with an upper respiratory tract infection. Where the discharge is constant from a central perforation the surgeon should suspect coincidental disease in the mastoid air cell system or the paranasal sinuses.
3. Social indications. Patients, particularly swimmers, may request repair of an ear drum to reduce the risks of infection. Some individuals may present with a symptomless perforation that has been detected on a pre-employment medical. If employment depends on the repair of such a perforation then it is reasonable to undertake surgery.

Pre-operative considerations

Many factors affect the likelihood of operative success. These include:

1. Site and size of the perforation.
2. Whether the perforation is central or marginal.
3. Frequency of aural discharge or infection.
4. The surgical technique used.
5. The material used to repair the ear drum.

Most surgeons would expect a success rate of over 90% for a small, dry central perforation. A marginal perforation that discharges frequently has a much lower operative success rate.

If a repair breaks down after surgery, a second operation may be successful if it is accompanied by a cortical mastoidectomy. Any paranasal sinus infection should be identified and treated.

A moist perforation may be accompanied by inflammation in the air cell system of the mastoid. In this case a cortical mastoidectomy performed at the same time as the myringoplasty may increase the chance of success.

If the Eustachian tube is blocked, although the graft may 'take', an effusion may occur. If there is some Eustachian tube function then increasing the size of the middle ear cleft by performing a cortical mastoidectomy may reduce the chance of development of a post-operative effusion.

Risks

Fortunately serious complications arising from a simple myringoplasty are rare. They include:

1. Failure of the graft to 'take'. This is usually due to infection or poor surgical technique.
2. Allergic reaction to the dressings.
3. Reduction in hearing. This may result from damage to the ossicular chain. If the ossicular chain is fixed and thus acts as a baffle to sound waves impinging on the round window, the hearing may reduce following a successful graft.
4. Trauma to the chorda tympani may affect taste. This is rarely a complaint.
5. Facial nerve palsy can occur, but is extremely rare. It is usually associated with a congenital abnormality. It has been hypothesized that trauma to the chorda tympani may lead to haemorrhage that tracks back into the facial nerve. It must be emphasized that facial palsy is virtually unheard of in myringoplasty surgery and rare in ossicular surgery.
6. Tinnitus occurs in most patients post-operatively. This problem usually settles as the ear heals.
7. Vertigo is very unusual unless the ossicles have been disturbed. A small portion of patients have vertigo following ossicular surgery, but this usually settles after 6 weeks. Major trauma to the inner ear at surgery may lead to severe post-operative vertigo, but this usually resolves in a matter of weeks unless the patient is elderly, when the unsteadiness may persist.

Preparation

The operation can be performed under either local or general anaesthesia. The ear is prepared and draped. There should be a foot-down tilt on the table. Running suction, operating microscope and drill should be available.

Method

1. The perforation is inspected. If a permeatal approach is to be used the whole margin of the perforation must be visible. With a permeatal approach the temporalis fascia graft is taken through a separate incision. The authors prefer an endaural approach as it gives good access and the graft can be taken via the same incision. A post-aural approach is used to combine the myringoplasty with a cortical mastoidectomy.
2. The edges of the perforation are excised using a needle and fine cupped forceps. The 'postage stamp' technique is shown in Figure 8.1.

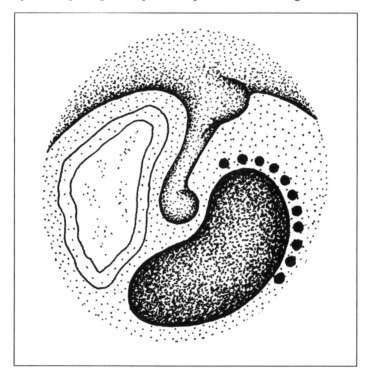

Figure 8.1   Preparation of the edge of a central perforation

3. Tympanosclerotic plaques in the drum should be removed. Small plaques can be excised with the drum. Larger plaques are more difficult to handle. The superficial layer of the drum is incised at the edge of the plaque and gently peeled off the plaque. Then a 'frying pan' type knife is passed between the plaque and the deep layer of the drum. Once freed the plaque is lifted out. In this manoeuvre the leaves of the drum are frequently damaged and torn. This is rarely a problem as long as the fascia graft underlies the traumatized area. Occasionally dense plaques anchor the ossicles to the surrounding bone. Violent manipulation of these plaques can lead to inner ear damage, so in this situation the surgeon may wish to separate the incudostapedial joint. When there is tympanosclerosis the mobility of the ossicular chain may be reduced due to ossicular fixation.

4. A posterior tympanomeatal flap is raised.
5. The temporalis fascia graft is cut to size. The graft should be large enough to cover the hole with a tail that is led up the posterior canal wall underneath the tympanomeatal flap. Some surgeons like the fascia to have been dried so that it is quite stiff prior to insertion. Other surgeons prefer the graft to be supple.
6. The graft is placed in the middle ear and deep to the tympanomeatal flap. The flap is returned to its position. Using two needles, the graft is manipulated so that the hole is closed. This is called the underlay technique. Occasionally the graft will not adhere to the deep surface of the drum. This occurs more often if the graft has been dried. When this happens the graft may need to be supported by finely chopped gel foam placed in the middle ear deep to the graft. There must be a complete seal between the margins of the perforation and the graft. The methods of graft placement are shown in Figure 8.2.

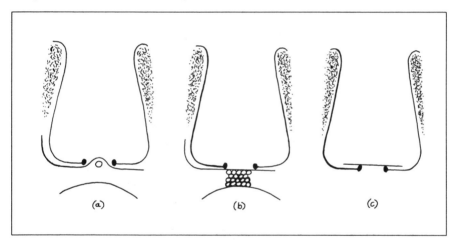

Figure 8.2 Variations in grafting technique: (a) Underlay technique with 'quilting' round the malleus long process. (b) Underlay technique supported with gel foam sponge. (c) Simple onlay technique

7. When the handle of the malleus is free it should be denuded of epithelium. The graft should normally be placed deep to the malleus. Sometimes the malleus handle has been pulled medially; there may even be an adhesion between the umbo and the promontory. In this situation any adhesions should be divided. To lateralize the handle of the malleus an osteotomy may be performed at the neck of the malleus. A malleus nipper can be used to fracture the malleus, but the handle should not be completely separated from the head. When the graft is inserted, it may lie on or very close to the promontory. In this situation there is a risk of adhesions forming between the graft and the promontory. To prevent this a sheet of 0.1 mm thick silastic is placed between the graft and the promontory.
8. Once the graft and flap are in their final position a thin sheet of silastic is laid over the drum and graft. The surface tension between the silastic and the graft helps to hold the graft in position. The authors then pack the

external auditory canal with cotton wool balls impregnated with bismuth iodoform paraffin paste. The endaural (or post-aural) incision is closed in two layers. A firm bandage is then placed over the ear to prevent haematoma formation.

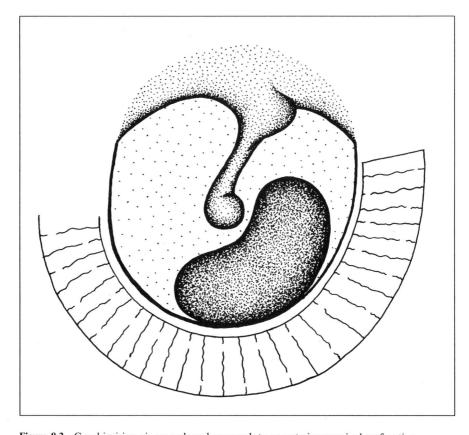

Figure 8.3   Canal incision via an endaural approach to an anterior marginal perforation

Modifications

1. Vein and dura can be used as a graft material. Dura is commercially available, but carries the risk of Creutzfeldt–Jakob disease.
2. The repair of an anterior perforation can be technically difficult. It can be difficult to get a good seal between the drum remnant and the graft. This is often compounded by poor visibility of the perforation due to the anterior meatal wall. Visibility of the anterior edge of the perforation may be improved by a post-auricular approach. Another alternative is to approach the anterior perforation with a prominent anterior meatal wall via an endaural incision. Then two parallel incisions are made in a circumferential fashion. Considering a right ear, the deep meatal incision is made about 1 mm from the annulus from 2 o'clock to 10 o'clock. The second parallel incision is made 5 mm from the annulus. The two incisions are joined at the

2 o'clock position. The incisions are shown in Figure 8.3. The flap is raised and rolled up. Great care should be taken in handling the flap. The flap is placed in the posterior half of the meatus and a piece of metal foil is placed over the flap to protect it. A diamond paste burr is then used to remove the bulge of the anterior wall and to improve visibility. Care should be taken not to enter the temporomandibular joint. The annulus is dislocated. A new deeper annular sulcus is drilled using a fine diamond burr. The graft is laid in and the drum remnant and flaps replaced.

Post-operative care

1. Immediately post-operatively the patient is nursed on his or her side with the operated ear uppermost. The pressure dressing is removed the following morning. Sutures are removed at 5 days.
2. The bismuth iodine paraffin paste (BIPP) impregnated dressings are removed between 2 and 3 weeks following surgery. Other types of dressing may need to be removed sooner.
3. Any middle ear blood clot has usually cleared by 6 to 10 weeks, when an audiogram should be performed.

OSSICULOPLASTY

Introduction

There are almost as many techniques as there are surgeons who perform this operation! Some basic tips are given here with a description of some of the techniques favoured by the authors.

Pre-operative considerations

Choice of prosthesis

Most surgeons favour using the patient's own tissues where possible. The range of possible materials are as follows:

1. Patient's own ossicles, removed and reshaped.
2. Cadaver ossicles.
3. Skull cortex (shaped).
4. Bone pate mixed with glue.
5. Septal or rib cartilage (often reinforced with wire).
6. Hydroxyl apatite commerically manufactured prostheses.
7. Ceramic or glass commercially manufactured prostheses.
8. Teflon or plastipore.

Human or bio-integratable materials are favoured because of the reduced risk of extrusion, especially when the implant is likely to be in direct contact with the ear drum. Many manufacturers recommend that bone pate or cartilage is placed between an artificial prosthesis and the ear drum.

The factors which determine whether an operation is likely to be successful are:

1. The nature and extent of ossicular damage. A simple disruption of the incudostapedial joint in the presence of an otherwise normal ossicular chain carries a very good prognosis. Extensive tympanosclerosis with fusion and fixation of all the ossicles carries a poor prognosis, even in the most skilled hands.
2. The skill of the surgeon.
3. Whether the ossiculoplasty is combined with a myringoplasty at the same operation. Combined surgery may reduce the success rate for the ossiculoplasty.
4. A history of frequent discharge reduces success rate.
5. Different prostheses carry different success rates.
6. Absence of the stapes superstructure is a poor prognostic sign.
7. Absence of the malleus, necessitating that the prosthesis must come in contact with the ear drum, reduces operative success.

Risks and preparation

See under myringoplasty.

Method

1. Initially the approach is the same as for myringoplasty. The authors favour an endaural approach. A posterior tympanomeatal flap is raised and the ossicular chain is examined.
2a. *Normal ossicular chain. Incudostapedial joint disrupted.* Where there is no ossicular erosion then a chip of cortical bone can be placed between the stapes head and the long process of the incus. Another alternative is to join the bones together with a little bone pate mixed with fibrin glue.

    If the long process of the incus is eroded then a piece of Teflon intravenous cannula may be used. The authors find that a size 17 FG is usually about right. A 4 mm length is cut and threaded over a straight needle and pushed down the shaft of the needle so as to stretch slightly one end. A small hole is then cut in the side of the tube about 1 mm from the narrow end. The tube is then slid over the incus (stretched end first) and the head of the stapes positioned in the hole.

    If most of the long process of the incus has been destroyed then the incus should be removed. It is usually removed easily, but if not the surgeon should suspect ossicular fixation. The incus is reshaped. A small pit is drilled in the head into which the stapes head will fit. The short process comes to lie under the neck of the malleus. A groove may be drilled in the short process to take the malleus as shown in Figure 8.4. The incus is reduced in size so that its centre of balance is the pit for the stapes. It is then placed in position. When the incus is severely eroded then an artificial prosthesis may be chosen. These are usually marked 'partial' to indicate that the stapes superstructure should be in place. They may be divided into two basic groups:

- Those which go between the stapes head and the malleus handle.
- Those which go between the stapes head and the ear drum. These prostheses are often too big and require shaping to fit. The manufacturer's instructions on shaping should be followed, but these are often inadequate. The authors prefer to hold the prosthesis between thumb and forefinger while shaping the prosthesis with a large diamond burr.

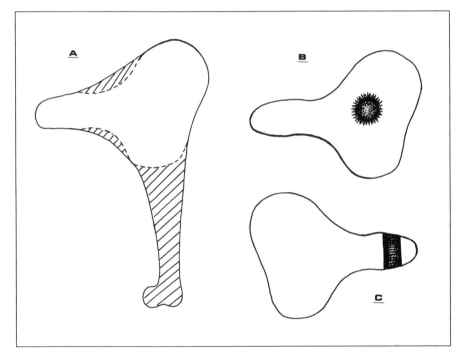

Figure 8.4 Incus: (a) prior to shaping; (b) after shaping showing the pit to hold the stapes' head; (c) after shaping showing the groove to hold the malleus' neck

Extrusion is minimized if the prosthesis is placed between the stapes and malleus handle. When this is not possible a stapes to drum assembly has to be used. In this situation the author prefers to use a prosthesis with a domed head made of hydroxyl apatite. First a temporalis fascia graft is placed under the drum at the point where the prosthesis will come into contact with the ear drum and then the prosthesis is inserted. If a ceramic material is chosen then a layer of bone pate should be placed on the head of the prosthesis. Extrusion is a particular problem with plastipore. To minimize this problem many surgeons recommend that a piece of septal cartilage is placed on the head of the prosthesis. Such plastic materials are now falling out of fashion.

2b. *Malleus and incus present but no stapes superstructure.* It is important to establish that the footplate of the stapes is mobile. If the footplate is fixed then either a small fenestra stapedotomy technique should be considered or the ear closed. N.B. If the footplate is mobile then the incus is removed. If there is sufficient length of the long process it can be used as an interposition between the malleus neck and the footplate. The incus is shaped like a crutch. The long process rests on the footplate and the head of the crutch is wedged under the neck of the malleus. A cadaver malleus may be used in a similar manner.

2c. *Mobile stapes footplate. Absent, fixed or abnormal malleus and incus.* Occasionally the malleus may be fixed and so a footplate to drum reconstruction has to be considered. These frequently fail due to:

- Extrusion.
- The prosthesis 'wanders' off the footplate.
- The prosthesis falls over.

Hydroxyl apatite prostheses, especially those with a domed head, appear to show some promise in this area. Nevertheless the prosthesis is not stable when standing on the footplate. A piece of fascia placed under the drum and a little fibrin glue dabbed on top of the prosthesis prior to insertion does facilitate a semi-stable assembly at surgery.

When all that is left is stapes footplate then a cadaver assembly of ossicles and drum may be implanted. Such cadaver assemblies are expensive to collect and maintain. The preservation methods may have long-term detrimental effects on the ossicles and their joints such that a conductive hearing loss develops over the post-operative period.

3. Once the ossiculoplasty has been performed the ear is closed in the same way as for a myringoplasty.

Tips on ossiculoplasty technique

1. When shaping the prosthesis try to avoid repeated insertions and removals. This keeps surgical interference of the stapes to a minimum. One way of doing this is to use measuring rods of silastic cut to different lengths.

2. If the prosthesis is slightly too big it is always tempting to wedge it into place. In doing this the stapes footplate may be forced into the inner ear or the malleus lateralized.

3. The ear drum is inclined medially from posterior to anterior. A stapes to drum assembly may give a situation where the anterior edge of the prosthesis is tenting the drum laterally. As time passes the portion of drum in contact with the anterior edge of the prosthesis fails and extrusion may result. To prevent this the anterior edge of the domed head of the prosthesis should be thinned or else a malleable headed prosthesis can be implanted.

4. Whenever possible the patient's own tissues should be used.

5. Many artificial materials such as hydroxyl apatite, ceramic and glass are very brittle. They will easily shatter when shaping if they are held with an instrument. A diamond paste burr is usually the best tool for shaping such implants.

Post-operative care

This is the same as for a myringoplasty. Some surgeons like to prescribe a prophylactic antibiotic.

The authors do not advise return to heavy manual labour for about 6 weeks, but those in sedentary jobs can return to work in the week following surgery.

EXCISION OF A GLOMUS TYMPANICUM TUMOUR

Introduction

A glomus tympanicum or paraganglioma of the middle ear is suspected by the appearance on otoscopy of a cherry red tumour behind the middle ear. Occasionally this tumour may present with aural bleeding. It is important to differentiate the tumour from a glomus jugulare. This is done by computerized tomography. Coronal cuts should reveal that the bone over the jugular bulb is intact and that there is air in the hypotympanum between the tumour and the jugular bulb. The operation is usually successful provided the diagnosis is correct. The oval window area may merely be involved with destruction of the stapes and when this occurs the complication rate is higher.

Risks

1. Misdiagnosis of a glomus jugulare tumour may lead to torrential haemorrhage requiring prompt packing of the ear and abandonment of the procedure. Packing will usually stop the bleeding but urgent embolization or ligation of the external carotid artery may rarely be required.
2. Misdiagnosis of a facial nerve neuroma may lead to paralysis of the face following surgery.
3. Conductive deafness due to ossicular damage.
4. Sensorineural deafness.
5. Facial palsy.
6. Vertigo if the inner ear is traumatized.
7. Tinnitus. This is usually present pre-operatively, but its nature may change if the inner ear is damaged..

Preparation

The patient is prepared as for a myringoplasty.

Method

1. An endaural incision is advised to improve access.
2. A posterior tympanomeatal flap is raised.

3. Great care should be taken when lifting the ear drum from the tumour. The tumour may be stuck to the tympanic membrane and start to bleed if handled roughly.
4. Once the tympanic membrane is elevated it is advisable to establish that the hypotympanum is free of tumour. An elevator or blunt dissector is passed round the tumour. In most instances these tumours arise from the promontory and once this has been established the tumour may be removed. A glomus tympanicum is friable and bleeds easily. It may be avulsed with granulation cupped forceps, while suction removes the blood to maintain vision of the working area. Once the tumour has been removed a small feeding artery is left bleeding on the promontory. Bipolar diathermy or a diamond burr can usually stop this haemorrhage.
5. A thin sheet of silastic is placed in the middle ear to prevent adhesions and the flap replaced.
6. The ear is dressed and the wound closed as for a myringoplasty.

Alternative methods

1. If an argon laser is available, then these highly vascular tumours can be shrunk or vaporized using this tool. Great care should be taken that the middle or inner ear structures are not heated excessively.
2. If a fine cryoprobe is used then the tumour can be frozen. The probe is placed on the tumour. Once the tumour has turned to an ice ball the probe is removed, bringing the tumour with it. Care should be taken that the tympanomeatal flap does not touch the cryoprobe or it will adhere.

Post-operative care

As for a myringoplasty.

TYMPANIC NEURECTOMY AND CHORDA TYMPANECTOMY

Indications

This procedure is used to treat Frey's syndrome or gustatory sweating which most commonly follows parotid surgery. This operation does markedly reduce gustatory sweating in many patients. The initial success that occurs in most patients is relatively short lived and by 2 years over 90% of patients will have relapsed. Even so, although the symptoms have returned many patients report considerable reduction in symptom severity.

Risks

As the ear drum and ossicles are likely to be normal, risks of this procedure are very small. The risks must include, however, conductive or sensory deafness, vertigo, tinnitus and facial palsy, as for any tympanotomy. Alteration in the sensation of taste to the tongue is common.

Preparation

The patient is prepared as for a myringoplasty.

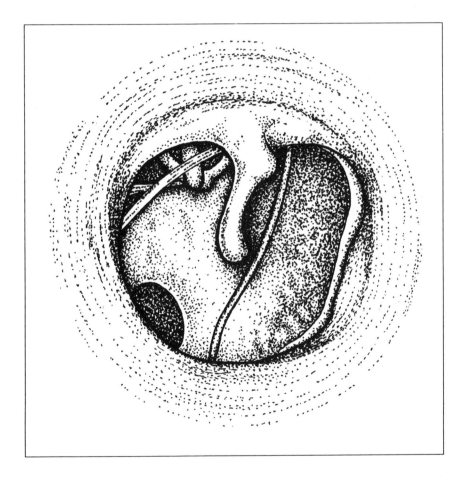

Figure 8.5 Illustration to show the course of the main branches of the tympanic plexus and the chorda tympani

Method

1. The operation can usually be performed via the meatus, but occasionally an endaural incision may be required for access.
2. A posterior tympanomeatal flap is raised. It is important that the annulus

is dislocated inferiorly round into the antero-inferior quadrant so that a good view of the promontory is obtained.

3. The chorda tympani is dissected free with a needle between the posterior wall and where it disappears from view between the incus and malleus. A 3–4 mm length of chorda is removed with the use of microscissors.

4. Coursing from postero-inferior to superior over the promontory, the two main branches of the tympanic plexus can usually be easily seen. This is shown in Figure 8.5. The mucosa over the promontory is removed. The two nerves are removed from the bony gutters in which they lie. At the inferior end they disappear into a bony canal. A diamond burr can be used to obliterate the entrance to this canal. The diamond burr can then be passed over the promontory several times to remove any nerve remnants and the middle ear irrigated to wash out any debris. Prior to using the burr a thin piece of metal foil should be laid over the flap of ear drum to protect it from the drill.

5. The tympanomeatal flap is replaced. The ear is dressed as for a myringoplasty.

Post-operative care

As for a myringoplasty.

Chapter 9

Stapedectomy

INTRODUCTION

Prior to the development of stapedectomy, the principal treatment for otosclerosis was a fenestration operation of the lateral semicircular canal. This necessitated the formation of a mastoid cavity. These cavities frequently became infected.

In 1958 Shea reported a stapedectomy technique using a vein graft over the oval window and a polythene strut. By the early 1960s various stapedectomy prostheses had been developed and the era of stapedectomy surgery was born. In those early days, as there was a large reservoir of untreated patients with otosclerosis, stapedectomy became one of the commonest ear operations, thus surgeons in those days developed great experience with many otologists doing over 100 operations per year. In the early 1980s the backlog of cases in the UK had been cleared and consequently otologists in training were finding it difficult to gain experience in this field of surgery.

At the same time as otologists were doing less stapedectomy surgery, the rise in medical litigation was on the way. This has led to a situation in which stapedectomy is now one of the commonest ear operations involved in litigation. Consequently the profession is beginning to respond by suggesting that only certain otologists perform stapes surgery. Thus experience is concentrated in the hands of one surgeon in any particular area. Certainly the occasional stapedectomy surgeon performing only two or three operations per year is more likely to run into problems. Another technique employed in some departments is to arrange stapedectomy surgery in batches every few months. By the time the surgeon is doing his or her third operation in a week he or she has become more adept and therefore is less likely to run into a problem with which he or she cannot cope expertly.

INDICATIONS

One of the reasons why surgery has become a less popular means of treating the conductive hearing loss found in otosclerosis is the advance made in hearing aid technology. Most patients in the UK are now offered a hearing aid as first choice of management. Many patients accept the aid as the quality and cosmetic appearance is much improved compared with what was available in the 1960s.

The primary indication for stapedectomy is a conductive hearing loss due to fixation of the stapes footplate. When the hearing in the other ear is normal then the patient needs to be carefully counselled. The risks of surgery should be measured against the possible gains and the patient allowed to decide without any pressure. In most instances, however, the hearing loss is bilateral and the operation should be performed on the worse ear. If there is a large sensori-neural component to the hearing loss then surgery may not be worthwhile as the patient may still require a hearing aid.

Contra-indications to stapedectomy

1. The patient is unfit for surgery due to other disease.
2. Age. Stapedectomy in the elderly is associated with a reduction in the speech discrimination post-operatively. However, excellent results have been reported in those over 70 years of age.
3. Children. The deafness is likely to be due to congenital fixation of the footplate and stapedectomy in this situation is associated with a high incidence of post-operative sensorineural deafness.
4. Stapedectomy should not be combined with other forms of ossicular manipulation at the same operation. A staged procedure gives good results.
5. The presence of external otitis or otitis media.
6. A stapedectomy should not be performed at the same time as a myringo-plasty.
7. In early cases where the audiometric handicap is minimal, say with a hearing loss less than 35 dB.
8. On the only hearing ear unless that ear is useless with a hearing aid.
9. Where there is a significant sensory deafness such that the patient would derive little or no benefit from the operation.
10. Stapedectomy should not be performed on an ear which appears to be affected by endolymphatic hydrops. However, if the patient has benign positional vertigo then the operation can be performed on the affected ear.
11. It may be unwise to operate on a patient whose occupation involves severe physical strain as there could be a risk of perilymph fistula.
12. In view of the risk of late sudden sensorineural deafness an operation on the second ear should be considered most carefully.

Risks

1. Sudden immediate sensorineural deafness. This, usually, occurs most often in the first few operations that the surgeon performs as he or she learns the technique. The incidence may be as high as 5% in the first 100 operations, but thereafter this drops to below 2% for most surgeons.
2. Delayed sudden sensorineural deafness. The aetiology of this is frequently unknown. Described causes include infection, barotrauma and necrosis of

the long process of the incus such that the prothesis penetrates the vestibule.

3. Vertigo. This is common immediately following surgery and can last for several days. It is due to minimal escape of perilymph around the prosthesis. The problem settles as healing takes place. Vertigo may persist if a perilymph fistula does not heal, necessitating a revision operation to plug any leak. Major trauma to inner ear structures may lead to a total loss of hearing with persistent vertigo. In this instance the vertigo is usually rotatory in nature, but gradually settles over a period of weeks. The patient who has lost labyrinthine function often has persistent unsteadiness, especially in the dark or on sudden head movement. Perilymph flooding may rarely occur at the time of surgery. This is believed to be associated with a congenital abnormality such as a wide cochlear aqueduct or direct communication with the internal auditory canal. The leak should be plugged. Sometimes insertion of a spinal drain and mannitol is required to allow the surgeon to plug the leak. The patient is usually left with a 'dead' ear.

4. Tinnitus. This is frequently relieved by a successful stapedectomy, but it may occur at any time post-operatively. The occurrence could be due to the development of cochlear otosclerosis. Tinnitus is a common cause of complaint in the patient who totally loses his or her hearing.

5. Facial palsy. This is fortunately rare. The facial nerve is at particular risk if it is dehiscent. Care should be taken to identify congenital abnormalities prior to manipulation of the footplate. These abnormalities include a facial nerve that overhangs the footplate or which splits round the posterior crus. If the nerve obscures the footplate then a stapedectomy should not be undertaken.

6. Infection. If the patient has an infection then the operation should be postponed. The surgeon should not operate if he or she is unwell.

Pre-operative considerations

Probably the most important single operative factor is the experience of the surgeon. As a guide the average surgeon, having performed less than 100 procedures, would expect to achieve a marked improvement in hearing in about 80–93% of cases; a severe sensorineural loss in about 4% and about 5–15% failure to close the air bone gap but without a significant sensorineural loss. Experienced surgeons will approach a 95% success rate.

PREPARATION

There are many different techniques, but one method favoured by MRH is described here.

The patient is prepared as for a myringoplasty. The pinna is cleaned with aqueous antiseptic, but the external auditory canal is only wiped clean with cotton wool. Some surgeons prescribe prophylactic penicillin before surgery commences.

METHOD

1. A small endaural incisions is made and the external canal held open with two, two-pronged self-retaining retractors.
2. A posterior tympanomeatal flap is raised and the middle ear entered.
3. The mobility of the ossicular chain is established and a fixed footplate confirmed.
4. The chorda tympani is dissected free with a needle and moved inferiorly. If the nerve will not move inferiorly without stretching then it is cut cleanly.
5. A sharp curette is used to remove bone from the posterior superior bony margin to give adequate exposure of the incudostapedial joint, footplate and facial nerve just above the footplate. The stapedial pyramid should be visible. The exposure is shown in Figure 9.1.

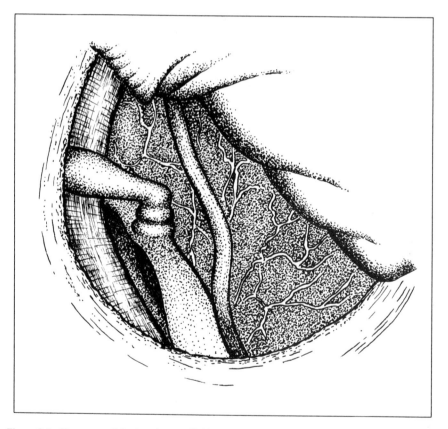

Figure 9.1   Exposure of the incudostapedial joint, stapes footplate and chorda tympani prior to stapedotomy

6. A measuring rod is used to measure the distance between the footplate and the incus. This distance is usually 4.5 mm. A 7 mm × 0.4 mm Teflon and platinum wire prosthesis is then mounted in a cutting block (MRH

uses that designed by Fisch). The prosthesis is cut to size and placed ready for placement in the ear.

7. If there is adequate access then the footplate should be perforated at this point of the operation; if not, the stapes superstructure should be removed.

8. With the stapes superstructure still in place, a 0.3 mm hand drill is used to penetrate the footplate. The hole is enlarged using a 0.4 mm and a 0.5 mm hand drill.

9. The prosthesis is then placed in position with the hook over the incus and the barrel of the prosthesis in the hole. It is important to ensure that the barrel does not catch on the edge of the fenestra. Using a crimper, the wire is secured round the incus long process. This is shown in Figure 9.2.

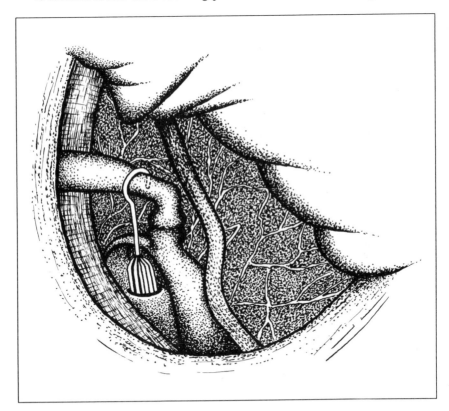

Figure 9.2 Prosthesis in place with the stapes superstructure still to be removed

10. The crura of the stapes are then removed using crura nippers. If possible the head of the stapes with the stapedial tendon should be left in place. The mobility of the assembly is tested by moving the malleus.

11. The prosthesis is usually such a snug fit that any leak round it ceases by placing a drop of blood on the footplate. However, should there be a leak several small pieces of fat can be placed round the barrel to secure a seal.

12. The flap is replaced and several pieces of gel foam placed as a dressing.

13.   The endaural incision and dressings are applied as for a myringoplasty.

Modifications of technique

1.   Placing the prosthesis prior to removal of the superstructure is difficult. Its main advantage is incus stability during placement and crimping of the prosthesis.

   The stapes superstructure can be removed first and then the footplate perforated (Figure 9.3). The prosthesis is now positioned. In this situation the incus is prone to 'wiggle' when trying to crimp the wire. There are two ways round this. One is to hold the incus stable with a second instrument or to use an all-Teflon prosthesis. The hook has a 'memory' (Figure 9.4). After the all-Teflon prosthesis is opened the hook begins to close. The prosthesis is placed immediately and gradually the hook closes round the long process of the incus. There is a risk with this type of prosthesis that as time passes the incus will necrose and the prosthesis disarticulate.

2.   The techniques described above may be considered as 'open' techniques in that the prosthesis itself is placed directly in fenestra. A major variation in technique is when the fenestra is first closed with a vein graft prior to placement of the prosthesis. This has the added advantage of sealing the inner ear and so reducing the risk of a perilymph leak. In this method the fenestra has to be significantly wider and usually a 0.8 mm fenestra is created.

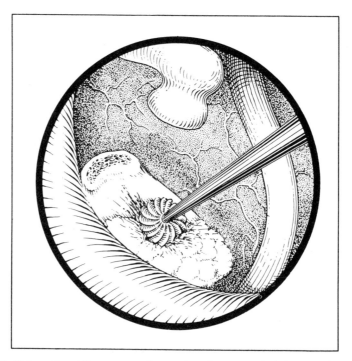

Figure 9.3   Using a fine drill to create a fenestration after removal of the stapes superstructure (from RSE, by permission)

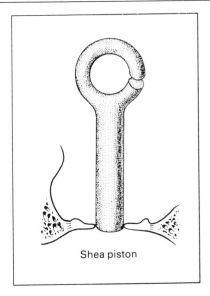

Shea piston

Figure 9.4 The all-Teflon prosthesis with a 'memory' (from RSE, by permission)

Special intra-operative situations

1. If a dehiscent facial nerve obscures the footplate then it is wiser to abandon the operation. When an intact facial nerve canal overhangs the footplate then usually an adequate view can be achieved by altering the angle of vision.
2. Bleeding. Every attempt should be made to control haemorrhage prior to opening the vestibule. Close co-operation between the surgeon and anaesthetist combined with foot-down tilt on the table are essential.
3. Floating footplate. If the footplate mobilizes before the vestibule is penetrated and the superstructure removed then the operation should be abandoned. If the footplate is intact and the superstructure has been removed then a prosthesis can be inserted between the floating footplate and the incus, thus achieving a good result. If the footplate is open but the hole is not large enough then it can be tilted by pressing gently on one crural attachment whilst insinuating a fine hook into the hole to remove a fragment. Repeated instrumentation should be avoided and if necessary the fenestra should be plugged and the operation abandoned.
4. The footplate should not be removed totally as a suction effect may disrupt the membranous labyrinth.

POST-OPERATIVE CARE

1. The patient should receive prophylactic antibiotics such as penicillin.
2. The patient is initially nursed lying on the side with the operated ear uppermost. As any vertigo subsides the patient is gradually sat up and

mobilized. This may be often within 24 hours, but some patients may require a slower mobilization regime.

3. Any anti-emetic is usually given by regular injection for the first 24 hours.

Management of complications

1. Infection should be treated promptly with a broad spectrum antibiotic.
2. Post-operative granuloma usually occurs between the third and tenth day. The patient complains of discomfort, vertigo and progressive hearing loss. Urgent exploration is warranted to remove the granuloma and seal the oval window.
3. Perilymph fistula is usually suspected because of persistent vertigo and hearing loss. These symptoms may be fluctuant if the leak is small. They merit re-exploration and plugging of the leak.
4. Failure to close the air bone gap or late onset of a conductive loss may be due to a slipped piston, necrosis of the incus, failure to crimp adequately, other fixed ossicles, or too short a prosthesis. Revision surgery has a poor success rate (around 50%). The vestibule should never be reopened as this carries a very high rate of sensorineural loss. Myringoplasty after stapedectomy has a 20% risk of inner ear damage.

Chapter 10

Mastoid surgery

INTRODUCTION

Mastoid surgery is the mainstay of treatment for chronic suppurative otitis media with or without cholesteatoma formation. A mastoidectomy may be considered:

1. To eradicate disease within the mastoid portion of the petrous temporal bone.
2. As a posterior or superior approach to the structures of the middle ear.
3. As a means of access to the structures of the inner ear, endolymphatic sac, internal auditory canal and cerebellopontine angle.
4. For access to the facial nerve.
5. To facilitate insertion of a cochlear implant.
6. To provide access to the jugular bulb and intrapetrous carotid artery.
7. As the initial part of a route to the petrous apex.
8. As an approach to the lateral end of the Eustachian tube.

CORTICAL MASTOIDECTOMY

Indications

1. Removal of diseased bone and air cells of the mastoid.
2. As an approach to the endolymphatic sac, semicircular canals, lateral venous sinus and dura over the anterolateral surface of the cerebellum.
3. To improve aeration of the middle ear cleft.
4. As part of a combined approach tympanoplasty. A cortical mastoidectomy is performed, then a posterior tympanotomy in which bone immediately lateral to the descending portion of the facial nerve is removed, thus cutting a 'window' from the cortical mastoid cavity into the mesotympanum without excising the entire posterior external auditory canal wall. This can give access to the round window for insertion of a cochlear implant electrode without disturbing the ear drum and external auditory canal.

The commonest reason for exploring the mastoid air cell system is suspected disease in the air cells and bone. Acute mastoiditis is now a rare condition in the UK, but 35 years ago was the commonest reason for performing a cortical mastoidectomy. The surgeon should suspect infected mastoid air cells in patients with a central tympanic perforation that chronically discharges (tubotympanic disease), especially after other sources of sepsis such as chronic sinusitis have been excluded. In this situation a cortical mastoidectomy accompanied by systemic antibiotics may achieve a dry ear such that a myringoplasty could be considered at a second stage procedure. Occasionally a chronic discharging ear with a central perforation may harbour a cholesteatoma. This will almost certainly be discovered when performing a cortical mastoidectomy. Cholesteatomas are more commonly associated with a posterior marginal or attic perforation.

Pre-operative considerations

1. It is impossible to discuss, other than in the most general terms, the success rates for a cortical mastoidectomy because the indications are so variable.
2. Cortical mastoidectomy for acute mastoiditis when coupled with systemic antibiotics nearly always settles the infection. In fact most of the complications of acute mastoiditis arise prior to surgery and are often associated with delayed presentation. Once the abscess is drained then resolution is usually rapid. If the patient presents with extensive intracranial venous thrombosis, meningitis or intracranial sepsis the prognosis can be significantly altered.
3. The patient with chronic tubotympanic disease is more difficult to manage and to achieve a dry ear. Cortical mastoidectomy is only part of this management. An attempt should be made to eradicate all sources of sepsis in the head and neck, especially dental and sinus sepsis. Diseased mucosa with polyp formation should be removed from the mesotympanum and especially from around the Eustachian tube orifice, if necessary via a tympanotomy. A cortical mastoidectomy should be performed and as many diseased air cells removed as possible. This surgery should be combined with a course of systemic antibiotic chosen as the result of bacteriological investigations. This usually achieves a dry ear. However, as months pass episodes of aural discharge return in an increasing number of patients. If the ear remains dry for about 3 months then a myringoplasty can be performed. This does reduce the relapse rate. Relapse is usually associated with a recurrence of upper respiratory infection. Certain groups nearly always relapse and include those who suffer from:

   • Nasal polyposis.
   • Atopy.
   • Mucociliary disorders.

4. Cholesteatoma recurrence following combined approach tympanoplasty (CAT) is very high. The main advantage of a combined approach tympanoplasty is the avoidance of a mastoid cavity. If a CAT is performed then a

'second look operation' is advisable about a year later to exclude residual cholesteatoma.

Risks

The risks for all mastoid surgery will be described here:

1. Sensorineural hearing loss. If any portion of the inner ear is inadvertently entered then a sensory hearing loss can result. If the stapes or any part of an intact ossicular chain is touched by a rotating burr the vibration can transmit damage to inner ear structures. Clearing cholesteatoma or diseased mucosa from around the stapes can also result in hearing loss. Occasionally disease has eroded the bone of the inner ear and this most commonly occurs over the lateral semicircular canal. Removing such disease may open the inner ear, leading to hearing loss.
2. Infection may arise post-operatively. This can spread to the inner ear, causing a suppurative labyrinthitis. The resultant symptoms include vertigo, deafness and tinnitus.
3. Conductive hearing loss. This is most often caused intentionally. It is usual to remove the incus and often the malleus head when a cholesteatoma is excised. Consequently a conductive hearing loss will result. This loss may be reduced by some form of ossicular reconstruction.
4. Vertigo is relatively uncommon following mastoid surgery. When there is an open cavity, cold winds blowing into the cavity may induce vertigo. If the inner ear is opened at surgery acute rotatory vertigo will result. This usually settles after a few days, but the patient is often left with a sensation of unsteadiness in the dark or on sudden head movement. Benign paroxysmal positional vertigo has been reported following mastoid surgery, but is very rare in this situation.
5. The facial nerve may be damaged. This may occur if the surgeon is unfamiliar with the anatomy of the ear and gets 'lost' within the mastoid. The facial nerve may rarely be in an ectopic position and, therefore, be encountered unexpectedly. Dehiscence of the facial nerve can occur. This is most commonly found just superior to the oval window. Peeling cholesteatoma matrix off the nerve at this point may bruise a dehiscent nerve. Facial palsy following mastoid surgery does not necessarily indicate negligence, especially in the situation of a dehiscent or congenitally abnormal course.
6. The dura may be inadvertenly opened giving a CSF leak. This rarely causes a problem. A temporalis fascia graft placed over the tear and held in place with a pack effects a seal. The leak may rarely continue, but insertion of a spinal drain, bed rest and fascial repair will close nearly all leaks.
7. The lateral sinus may be opened. The patient should be placed head down immediately to prevent air embolus. Fascia is placed over the hole and the insertion of a pack will stop the bleeding.

Preparation

The patient is prepared and draped as for the myringoplasty. Running suction, drill, operating microscope and adequate illumination are required.

Method

1. The postauricular skin is infiltrated with a vasoconstrictor solution. A postauricular incision is made and the mastoid bone exposed (see Chapter 8).
2. The surface marking of the antrum is MacEwen's triangle just postero-superior to the spine of Henle. In the adult the antrum is about 1.5 cm from the surface, but can be considerably less in children. An impression of the size of the mastoid air cell system may be obtained from a lateral radiograph.
3. Using the largest cutting burr available, the mastoid cortex is removed and the air cell system entered. The lateral sinus plate and dural plates are identified. Gradually the cavity is deepened working from deep to superficial with the burr. Bone is removed superficial to the antrum until the antrum is entered. This antrostomy is gradually widened. Using a blunt probe, the incus is gently palpated through the aditus. These landmarks are shown in Figure 10.1. The aditus is widened. The largest burr that will not damage adjacent structures should always be used.
4. When approaching inner ear structures, dura, lateral sinus or facial nerve a diamond paste burr should be used. When approaching the dense bone of the otic capsule and Fallopian canal the surgeon will notice a change in colour to dense bone with a yellowish tinge. A 'tinny' or change in the sound of the drill occurs as the surgeon approaches dura or the lateral sinus plate. Frequent washing of the cavity will help to remove any blood and simplify the identification of important landmarks. Once the incus has been identified the bone of the posterior canal wall can be thinned. Air cells should be removed from the mastoid tip, root of zygoma and the occipital bone. The mastoid tip need not be removed unless it is necrotic. The sinodural angle should be clearly defined. If granulations are encountered on the dura then the dura should be exposed until healthy dura is encountered. Any extradural abscess should be drained into the cavity. Any pus encountered in the procedure should be sent for bacteriological examination.
5. Occasionally masses of granulation tissue may be encountered. If the surgeon suspects that vital structures may have been exposed by this disease then great care must be taken. Normal anatomy should be clearly identified away from the granulation tissue and planes of dissection should be gradually opened working from normal anatomy into the diseased area.
6. A tube drain is placed into the cavity if any infection has been encountered and the wound closed in layers with interrupted sutures. A pressure bandage is applied.

Post-operative care

1. In infected cases antibiotics should be continued for a full course. In acute mastoiditis nasal decongestants are administered to facilitate middle ear aeration via the Eustachian tube.
2. The head bandage is removed the following day and the sutures removed in about 6 days.

3. Any drain is removed once discharge ceases. This usually occurs after about 3 days.
4. An audiogram is performed when the patient has recovered.

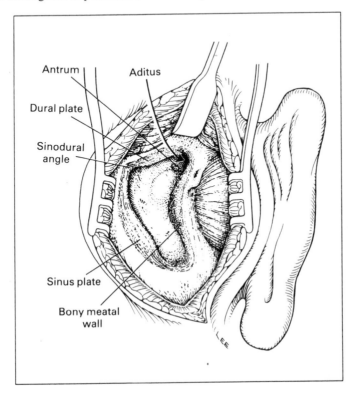

Figure 10.1 Landmarks of a cortical mastoid cavity (from RSE, by permission)

POSTERIOR TYMPANOTOMY

Indications

1. To gain access to the mesotympanum via the cortical mastoid cavity.
   - This route may be used to insert a cochlear implant, in which case the external auditory canal is left undisturbed.
   - A posterior tympanotomy may be combined with an approach via the external auditory canal to excise diseased mucosa, cholesteatoma and facilitate an ossicular reconstruction without 'taking down' the posterior canal wall. This gives excellent access to the facial recess, but the sinus tympani is still hidden.

Method

1. A cortical mastoidectomy is performed.

2. The incus and digastric ridge are carefully identified. Thus the line of the facial nerve can be visualized. The area of bone removed is shown in Figure 10.2. Using a 1 mm diamond drill and plenty of irrigation, drilling is commenced immediately lateral to the line of the facial nerve and immediately inferior to the incus short process. Gradually a window is cut between the facial nerve medially and the annulus laterally. Consequently the stapes and round window can be seen through the mastoid cavity, as in Figure 10.3(a) and (b).

3. Great care must be taken not to damage the facial nerve. A facial nerve stimulator can be of value especially to distinguish between nerve and mucosa in an uncapped air cell. Care must be taken not to touch the stapes or ossicular chain with a rotating burr.

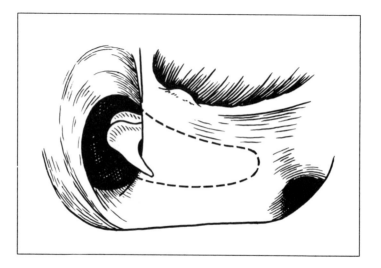

Figure 10.2   The dotted area shows the bone to be removed in a posterior tympanotomy (from RSE, by permission)

CANAL WALL DOWN MASTOIDECTOMY

Indications

1. Excisions of cholesteatoma.
2. Exploration of the mastoid portion of the facial nerve.
3. Excision of tumours involving the mastoid and jugular bulb.
4. Excision of granulomatous or mucosal disease.

Pre-operative considerations

It is important to define the surgical aims. In the case of cholesteatoma these are:

1. Prevention of intra-cranial complications.
2. Prevention of facial palsy, suppurative labyrinthitis and sensorineural hearing loss, with or without vertigo due to erosion of the inner ear.
3. To obtain a dry ear.
4. To maintain or restore hearing.

Complete excision of the cholesteatoma with exteriorization of the middle ear cleft usually achieves the first and second aims in most cases. Recurrence, however, of cholesteatoma is not uncommon. This disease may be relatively minor and easily controlled in the out-patient clinic by aural toilet. Occasionally a massive recurrence goes unnoticed and the patient then presents with one of the significant complications. For this reason regular, thorough inspection of the cavity on an annual basis is recommended.

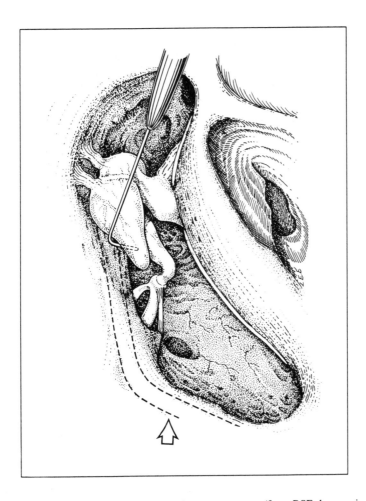

Figure 10.3(a) Structures revealed via a posterior tympanotomy (from RSE, by permission)

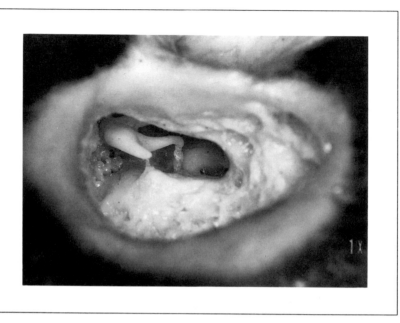

Figure 10.3 (b)   This right temporal bone dissection demonstrates the structures revealed via a posterior tympanotomy

A cavity that continues to discharge is very common. It may occur in as many as 30% of patients. The reasons for persistent discharge from a mastoid cavity include:

1. Inadequate meatoplasty.
2. Incomplete excision of cholesteatoma.
3. Exposed infected or oedematous mucosa within the cavity.
4. A poorly designed cavity, often with a high facial ridge.
5. Retained infected air cells.
6. Repeated contamination of the cavity with dirty water such as bath water.
7. Tympanum and Eustachian tube open to the exterior such that mucus may discharge into the cavity with upper respiratory infections.

Many patients with chronic otitis media have a mild sensorineural hearing loss. This cannot be corrected. The cholesteatoma itself can be an efficient conductor of sound in some circumstances so that when it is excised with any diseased ossicles the patient has a total conductive hearing loss unless a tympanoplastic procedure is performed. Even with a tymplanoplasty hearing is frequently not restored to pre-operative levels. The surgeon may not wish to consider a tympanoplasty, particularly if residual cholesteatoma remains in the oval window.

Mastoidectomy should be considered as a range of operations which merge into one another. The least radical operation is an atticotomy in which only the outer attic wall is removed. This can be extended backwards so that the aditus and antrum are exposed (atticoantrostomy). A further extension will open the air cell system proper of the mastoid, necessitating that the posterior meatal wall is excised. Finally the mesotympanum and hypotympanum may have to be exposed and if necessary the tympanic membrane excised in part or completely (modified radical or radical mastoidectomy).

Method

Atticotomy

1. The patient is prepared and draped as for a cortical mastoidectomy. The choice of incision depends on the extent of the disease. If the surgeon is confident that only an atticotomy is required then an endaural approach is reasonable. However, if a large cholesteatoma is suspected or it may be necessary to expose the mastoid tip a postaural approach is preferred.
2. A posterosuperior meatal skin flap is raised and reflected antero-inferiorly to expose the bone of the superior aspect of the external auditory canal. Using a 4 mm cutting burr and working from deep to superficial, the bone of the outer attic wall is thinned, thus widening the meatus superiorly (Figure 10.4).

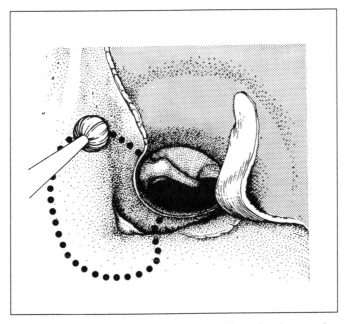

Figure 10.4   The dotted area shows the bone to be removed in performing an atticotomy (from RSE, by permission)

3. The annulus is dislocated and the tympanic membrane elevated to reveal the incudostapedial joint. The joint is disarticulated if ossicular continuity is present.
4. Using a 2 mm diamond burr, the outer attic wall is gradually removed to reveal the mucosa over the ossicular heads. If the cholesteatoma is entirely lateral to the ossicular heads and confined to the attic it is now removed (Figure 10.5).

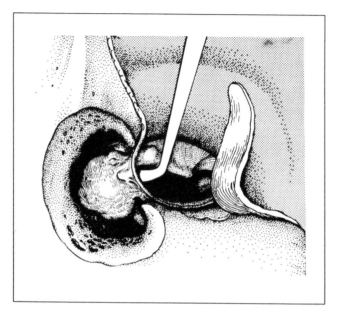

Figure 10.5   Cholesteatoma has been revealed in the attic surrounding the ossicular heads (from RSE, by permission)

5. If the cholesteatoma extends deep to the ossicular heads then they are carefully exposed by 'drilling out' the last of the outer attic wall. The incus is removed. The head of the malleus is removed using malleus shears (Figure 10.6). This exposes the medial attic wall. The pars tensa is mobilized to give an adequate view of the anterior attic and mesotympanum. Starting anteriorly, as the facial nerve is least likely to be dehiscent in this area, the cholesteatoma sac is carefully and thoroughly excised with the aid of a blunt dissector or elevator.
6. A temporalis fascia graft is harvested. A piece of conchal cartilage is obtained and carved to fill the defect in the outer attic wall (Figure 10.7). An ossiculoplasty is performed. This is usually a stapes to drum or footplate to drum assembly. Fascia is laid over the cartilage and underneath the tympanic membrane prior to placement of the ossicular prosthesis.
7. The skin flap is replaced. A thin silastic sheet is laid over the fascia and flap. The canal is packed. The wound is closed with interrupted sutures and the patient prescribed prophylactic antibiotics if the ear is infected.

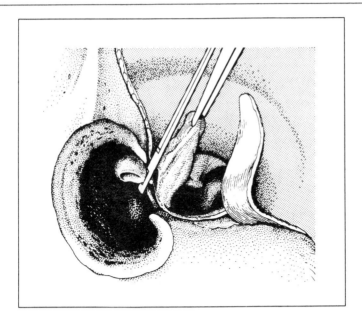

Figure 10.6 Excision of the head of the malleus to aid removal of cholesteatoma (from RSE, by permission)

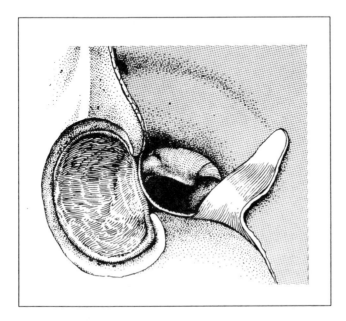

Figure 10.7 Reconstruction of the outer attic wall using temporalis fascia and conchal cartilage (from RSE. by permission)

Atticoantrostomy and mastoidectomy

1. An atticotomy is performed as in steps 1–4 above. The atticotomy is extended backwards uncovering the cholesteatoma. Gradually bone is removed working from deep to superficial. The mastoid air cell system is exenterated. The lateral sinus and dural plates are identified. The posterior meatal wall should not be lowered completely until the position of the facial nerve is ascertained. The sac is carefully elevated from a posterior direction (working anteriorly) until the lateral semicircular canal is identified (Figure 10.8). The surgeon now dissects the cholesteatoma backwards (posteriorly) from the anterior attic to identify and expose the facial nerve canal (Figure 10.9). The horizontal portion of the facial nerve is followed backwards. Portions of the cholesteatoma are excised as the dissection progresses. Cholesteatoma is peeled off the lateral semicircular canal. Eventually all the cholesteatoma is excised except for a small portion in the facial recess, oval window and possibly sinus tympani.

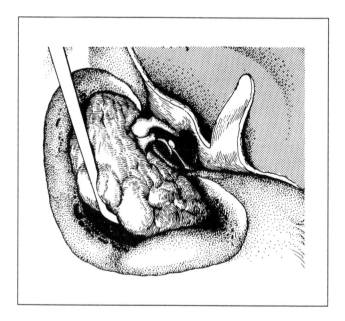

Figure 10.8   Elevation of the cholesteatoma from a posterior approach (from RSE, by permission)

2. Once the line of the facial nerve has been established the posterior meatal wall may be lowered to its final position. A large diamond burr (6 mm) is used with copious irrigation. The drill is worked in the line of the facial nerve and is always kept moving. This technique exposes the facial recess and oval window area. Using fine cupped forceps and elevators, any residual cholesteatoma matrix and sac is excised.

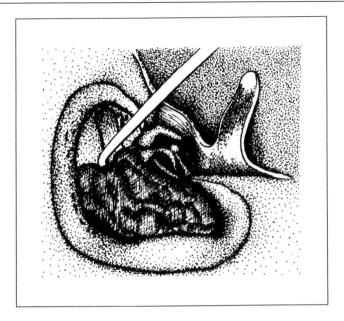

Figure 10.9 Elevation of the cholesteatoma from anterior to posterior to reveal the facial nerve

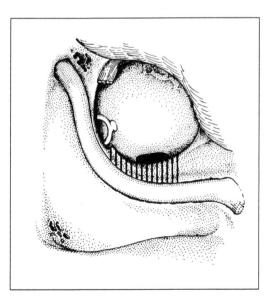

Figure 10.10 This shows the bone anterior to the facial nerve, which has to be removed in order to reveal the sinus tympani (from RSE, by permission)

3. If cholesteatoma is lying in the sinus tympani then bone may need to be removed from the anterior aspect of the nerve using a large diamond burr (Figure 10.10). Despite this manoeuvre adequate visibility may not be achieved. If this is the case, the patient's head may have to be turned

towards the surgeon so that he or she may view the sinus tympani from an anterior aspect to facilitate removal of the last of the cholesteatoma.

4. The cavity may now be polished and 'bowled'. If the mastoid tip is removed the soft tissues will collapse into the cavity in this area.

5. As much temporalis fascia as is reasonably possible should now be harvested. This fascia is placed under the tympanic membrane remnant and draped across the facial ridge. If the stapes superstructure is still present then a Type III reconstruction can be fashioned. Any remaining fascia is used to line the cavity. A thin silastic sheet is laid across the fascia to prevent any pack sticking to the graft.

6. A meatoplasty is fashioned (see Chapter 8).

7. An antiseptic pack such as bismuth iodine paraffin paste (BIPP) is inserted and the incision closed in layers.

8. A pressure head bandage is applied.

Post-operative care

1. The pressure bandage is usually removed after 24 hours. A drain is rarely required, but if a temporalis muscle flap has been raised then drain insertion is often advisable to prevent haematoma collection.

2. Prophylactic antibiotics are not usually required. The common infecting organisms in chronic suppurative otitis media are pseudomonas, proteus and bacteriodes. The excision of the cholesteatoma and the use of irrigation are probably important factors in preventing infection. However, if the dura is breached then antibiotics should be prescribed. An antibiotic active against pseudomonas should be chosen.

3. Immediately following surgery, facial movement should be inspected and noted.

4. Sutures are removed at 5–7 days. The BIPP pack may be left for several weeks. In young children it is usual to give a short general anaesthetic to remove the pack.

5. After removal of the pack the cavity is left open to the air. The patient is warned not to block the meatus with cotton wool. Good ventilation is important to achieve a dry healthy cavity. Any granulations in the cavity should be removed. Granulations that are well clear of the drum and facial nerve may be cauterized with silver nitrate.

6. An audiogram should be performed about 6 weeks after surgery.

7. Some patients are keen to swim. Each case should be judged on its own merit. Patients should never swim alone in case they become vertiginous from water entering the cavity. A purpose-made swimming plug with a tight bathing cap may afford adequate protection to permit swimming.

MANAGEMENT OF POST-OPERATIVE FACIAL PALSY

Immediate facial palsy

A facial palsy discovered when the patient is recovering from the general anaesthetic may be due to local anaesthetic that has been infiltrated prior to surgery. A total facial palsy present after recovery from anaesthesia indicates a major injury to the nerve. Occasionally such a palsy may not be unexpected, particularly if there is extensive exposure of the nerve by a cholesteatoma. In this situation the surgeon may have already decompressed the nerve knowingly and be confident of its integrity. In such a situation nothing more needs to be done other than making a careful record of the surgery and explaining the findings to the patient. If it is possible to photograph the findings during operation then this should be done.

When the palsy is unexpected then the nerve requires urgent exploration and decompression. Once the palsy has been found a careful explanation should be given to the patient, preferably with a witness present. If the surgeon is confident in the procedure of facial nerve decompression then the operation should be scheduled for the next available operating list. It is often advisable to ask a colleague to assist. This colleague can give an independent assessment of the findings at surgery which may be of value should litigation arise. If it is possible the exploration should be recorded on video or photographs taken of the operative findings.

As well as making meticulous notes of the extent of the palsy clinically, photographs of the patient should be obtained. Additional photographs may be taken as the facial palsy begins to recover.

Delayed facial palsy

This problem can be more difficult to manage. The most difficult decision is whether to decompress the nerve. As the facial movements were known to be normal following operation, the nerve must be in continuity. The nerve may be bruised or compressed by the pack. It is certain that the nerve is exposed. Usually the only action required is to remove the pack. EMG studies will reveal that there is little or no degeneration and recovery can be expected within 3 weeks.

The paralysis is rarely rapid in onset as a result of a haemorrhage within the nerve or a splinter of bone piercing the sheath. Usually the surgeon can recall in detail his or her actions close to the facial nerve and knows whether the possibility of an intra-neural injury exists. If the surgeon believes that an intra-neural injury may have taken place then a decompression should be performed. This will reduce the risk of intra-neural fibrosis and a poor return of nerve function. Should the surgeon decide against exploration then the nerve should be electrically monitored. Reduction in the combined action potential to less than 10% of the normal side within 6 days or the presence of denervation potentials on EMG, at 2 weeks, indicate a poor prognosis. Prompt decompression at this point may influence the final outcome.

Late presentation

Occasionally a surgeon may be asked to see a facial palsy case that has been managed conservatively and failed to recover.

Within the first 8 weeks of surgery if the palsy was of immediate onset following surgery, or there is presence of denervation potentials then prompt decompression is indicated.

Between 8 and 16 weeks from the time of surgery EMG should be performed weekly. The presence of polyphasic action potentials indicate reinervation. If there is still no recovery then the nerve should be explored. After one year exploration will rarely alter the nature of the facial palsy and other forms of facial reanimation should be considered.

MANAGEMENT OF THE DISCHARGING CAVITY

Unfortunately chronic aural discharge is a frequent complication of a mastoid cavity. Each case has to be carefully assessed and the factors preventing a dry ear corrected. Commonly encountered problems are as follows:

1. *Inadequate meatoplasty*

A large cavity requires a wide meatus for adequate ventilation. This problem may be solved by either obliterating the cavity or widening the meatus.

2. *Recurrent cholesteatoma*

This is surprisingly common. The recurrent cholesteatoma should be removed along with any diseased skin or granulation tissue. The cavity is then polished and relined.

3. *High facial ridge*

If the facial ridge is kept in place then granulation tissue or recurrent cholesteatoma can form in a mastoid bowl, which is inaccessible through the meatus. To prevent this problem the facial ridge should be lowered and the meatus widened.

4. *Granulation tissue in the cavity*

This usually arises when the cavity contains many uncapped air cells. The mucosa in these cells become infected and oedematous. This problem, there-fore, occurs most commonly in the well aerated mastoid. At revision surgery the air cells are exenterated and the cavity smoothed. This may require exposure of cells in the mastoid tip and as a consequence the cavity may become very large. To reduce the size of the cavity the facial ridge is lowered and the mastoid tip amputated. The soft tissues can then collapse into the inferior aspect of the cavity. Air cells that extend deep to the semicircular canals cannot be excised easily. This part of the air cells system may be sealed off from the cavity. A temporalis muscle flap can be rotated into the cavity and fascia used to line the reduced cavity and to cover the muscle flap.

If there is no cholesteatoma within the mastoid cavity then the posterior meatal wall can be reconstructed. The mastoid cavity is thoroughly cleaned of skin and granulation tissue, after which the cavity is polished. A piece of ceramic or hydroxyl apatite is fashioned to replace the posterior meatal wall. The prosthesis is glued in place. The meatal aspect of the new canal wall is covered with fascia which is led under the drum remnant. The meatus is packed. The packing is removed after 3 weeks.

5. *Granulation tissue in the oval or round windows*

This usually occurs if cholesteatoma sac has been left behind in these areas at initial surgery. It is not uncommon to find the ear drum remnant is perforated. This problem can be very awkward. Firstly, it may be impossible to remove safely any cholesteatoma sac without risk to the facial nerve or inner ear. Secondly, the facial nerve may be embedded in granulation tissue. Prior to admission it is useful to reduce any infection and oedematous mucosa by careful aural toilet in the out-patient clinic. A little local anaesthetic can be instilled into the cavity prior to removing the granulation tissue and if this technique produces a facial palsy then the surgeon can expect an exposed facial nerve in the cavity.

At surgery the horizontal facial nerve canal is identified at its anterior end. It is then followed backwards into the area of granulation tissue. The diseased tissue is carefully removed from the nerve canal. The polypoid mucosa is then removed from the oval window area. If indicated the facial ridge is lowered. At the level of the round window bone may be removed from the anterior aspect of the facial nerve canal to reveal the sinus tympani. The sinus tympani can then be cleared of diseased mucosa and cholesteatoma. The edges of the tympanic membrane are freshened and a temporalis fascia graft used to repair the ear drum. A thin sheet of silastic can be inserted into the middle ear to prevent adhesions and pocket formation.

6. *The intractably discharging cavity*

Occasionally the surgeon is presented with a cavity that despite revision surgery, antibiotics, and a diligent search for systemic causes such as Wegener's granuloma, continues to have a foul and incapacitating discharge. In this situation a total obliteration after subtotal petrosectomy can be considered.

The mastoid cavity is opened via a postauricular incision. The external auditory meatus is completely closed. All skin and mucosa in the cavity is totally excised. The following structures are skeletonized to ensure that as many air cells as possible are removed: the dura, the lateral sinus, the facial nerve, the inferior aspect of the cochlea and the semicircular canals. If diseased air cells or cholesteatoma extend into the petrous apex then the cochlea and semicircular canals should be removed. The orifice of the Eustachian tube is widened. The Eustachian tube is packed with muscle and sealed closed with bone wax. The large residual cavity is packed with fat harvested from the abdominal wall. The temporalis muscle is transposed inferiorly and stitched in place to obliterate the cavity. The skin flap is replaced and the wound closed. A drain may be required but should be removed as soon as possible. Prophylactic antibiotics are given for 48 hours. As the cavity is usually infected with pseudomonas the authors currently prescribe ticarcillin and clavulinic acid.

Although hearing is sacrificed by this technique, the few patients in whom this is necessary find this a small price to pay compared with offensive discharge and the repeated trips to hospital.

A CT scan should be performed at one, two and five years to exclude the development of a dermoid cyst within the temporal bone.

REVISION SURGERY FOR HEARING

It is not uncommon to find that no attempt has been made at a tympano-plasty at the initial mastoidectomy. When the patient has normal hearing in the other ear the results of ossicular reconstruction in a mastoid cavity are disappointing. It is often impossible to achieve a hearing level within 20 dB of the good ear; not least because of the frequent finding of coincidental sensori-neural loss. However, in the patient with bilateral suppurative otitis media then the surgery for hearing restoration can be very rewarding.

Preparation

The patient is prepared as for an ossiculoplasty. The cavity should be clean, dry and free from infection.

Method

1. Ideally there should be an aerated middle ear cleft roofed over by an intact tympanic membrane remnant. A small perforation of the remnant, however, may be repaired at the same time with a fascia graft.
2. Usually the malleus and incus are missing. Alternatively the handle of the malleus is the only ossicular remnant.
3. An incision is made down the facial ridge and continues onto the floor of the meatus. Care should be taken not to start the incision at the level of the second genu of the facial nerve lest the nerve be damaged.
4. The tympanomeatal flap is elevated and the middle ear entered at the meatal floor. The dissection is carefully continued superiorly until the stapes comes into view. The usual finding is of either an empty footplate only or an intact stapes.
5. When the stapes superstructure is present then a successful result is more likely. A hydroxyl apatite cap is placed on the stapes head and the flap replaced. If the drum is very thin then it should be reinforced with a fascia graft.
6. When there is a footplate only its mobility should be tested. If footplate fixation is found the procedure is abandoned. If the footplate is mobile then a piece of fascia is placed under the drum and a hydroxyl apatite total prosthesis is shaped to fit and inserted. If necessary it can be supported by a little piece of gel foam. It is important that the drum is not 'tented over' the prosthesis otherwise the likelihood of extrusion increases. The flap is replaced.
7. A thin sheet of silastic is placed over the drum and a pack placed in the cavity.

Additional points

Occasionally the surgeon is faced with a clean cavity but with absolutely no drum so that the Eustachian tube and both oval and round windows can be clearly seen. A graft laid diagonally across the cavity which seals off the round window and Eustachian tube from the rest of the cavity may increase the hearing by 20 dB. The hearing gain is rarely worth the effort of surgery in this situation.

Chapter 11

Surgery of the inner ear

INTRODUCTION

Surgery of the inner ear falls into three groups:

1. Destructive operations for vestibular problems.
2. Hearing preservation operations for vestibular problems.
3. Cochlear implantation to restore hearing in the post-lingually deafened patient.

1. The destructive operations for vestibular problems are membranous and osseous labyrinthectomy.
2. Since the 1920s a whole range of hearing preservation operations were developed to treat Meniere's disease. Decompression or drainage of the saccus endolymphaticus has gained tremendous popularity with a 60–80% success rate and a low complication rate. This is despite research performed in Copenhagen that appears to show that a cortical mastoidectomy is as effective as endolymphatic sac surgery.

    Cryotherapy and ultrasonic treatment to the inner ear have been advocated as a means of controlling Meniere's disease and maintaining hearing. In these techniques the lateral or even all three semicircular canals are exposed and the bone drilled until the 'blue line' of the canal is in view. Then either an ultrasonic or cryo-probe is applied. The patient is usually awake and nystagmus is observed. Initially the nystagmus is irritative in nature, but after a time changes direction to indicate paralysis of labyrinthine function. Although effective methods of treatment, neither technique has been widely accepted.

    The Fick sacculotomy and Cody tack sacculotomy, to treat Meniere's disease, had a brief spell of popularity in the mid 1960s. However, the dead ear rate for this procedure was unacceptably high and the operations fell into disrepute.

    Vestibular neurectomy is now an accepted effective treatment for severe Meniere's disease. Complications are, fortunately, unusual, but may be serious or fatal when they occur.

SURGERY OF THE ENDOLYMPHATIC SAC

Indications

Endolymphatic hydrops which is not controlled by medical treatment. This has to be interpreted for each individual. The elderly lady who gets mild attacks weekly may be happy on medical management, whereas the young fit man who gets severe attacks twice a year may accept an offer of surgery. Medical treatment would usually include betahistine, a diuretic, a reduced salt diet and an anti-emetic preparation.

Pre-operative considerations

Initially the relief of vertigo is in the order of 70–80%, but as time passes recurrence of vertigo becomes almost the rule. However, many patients find that if the vertigo does recur it is not as severe as before surgery and can be controlled by medication. If the operation is performed early in the course of the disease, especially if the hearing fluctuates, then there may be a post-operative improvement in the hearing. Tinnitus may also improve or disappear in a small percentage of cases following surgery.

Risks

Complications of this surgery are uncommon.

1. Sensorineural hearing loss. This can arise if infection occurs and spreads to the inner ear or if the ossicular chain is touched with a spinning burr. Inadvertent opening of the inner ear may lead to a dead ear, but provided that the fenestration is recognized at the time and plugged then this complication does not always follow.
2. Conductive hearing loss. The incus is really the only ossicle at risk in this operation. Trauma to the incus may lead to a conductive hearing loss.
3. Facial nerve palsy. The descending portion of the nerve may be encountered, particularly when searching for an inferiorly placed endolymphatic sac.
4. The dura may be breached – see Chapter 10.
5. The lateral sinus may be opened.

Preparation

1. The patient is prepared as for a cortical mastoidectomy.

Method

1. A cortical mastoidectomy is performed. The lateral sinus plate, dural plate and lateral semicircular canal should all be identified.

2. The endolymphatic sac is situated on the dura between the posterior semicircular canal and the lateral venous sinus. The sac runs from antero-superior to postero-inferior and it roughly bisects the angle between the line of the descending portion of the facial nerve and the line of the lateral semicircular canal.

3. A large cutting burr is used to remove the bone immediately anterior to the lateral venous sinus. Then a large diamond burr with copious irrigation is used to expose the dura. A periosteal elevator is used to remove the flakes of bone that may be adherent to the dura. This is shown in Figure 11.1. The dura is progressively separated from the bone with the use of the elevator until the sac is identified.

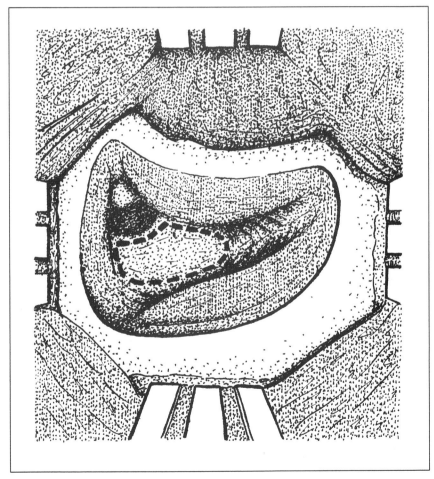

Figure 11.1   The dotted line shows the area of bone to be removed in order to expose the posterior fossa dura and endolymphatic sac. Right ear positioned on table

4. The sac can be difficult to find. Sometimes it is so fibrosed that it is little more than a white linear thickening of the dura. Occasionally the sac can be very short.
5. At this point there are many variations in surgical technique. Some surgeons only expose the sac while other surgeons may open the sac and insert a drain or a valve. Some surgeons suggest opening the medial wall of the sac.
6. The wound is closed in two layers and a pressure head bandage applied.

Post-operative care

1. The head bandage is removed the following day and the sutures at 5–7 days.
2. Post-operative facial movement is checked immediately after recovery.
3. The patients are rarely vertiginous after surgery, but an anti-emetic should be prescribed if required.
4. If the dura has been opened then prophylactic antibiotic may be prescribed. Some surgeons always prescribe antibiotics.
5. The patient is mobilized from the first post-operative day.

MEMBRANOUS LABYRINTHECTOMY

Indications

A peripheral labyrinthine dysfunction with poor hearing such as advanced Meniere's disease or other cause of endolymphatic hydrops. This operation may be used to control the vertigo that follows a stapedectomy with a total loss of hearing.

Pre-operative considerations

The success of the operation depends on a meticulous technique. Failure to control episodes of acute rotatory vertigo following surgery is rare. If functioning neuro-epithelium is left behind then there can be symptoms of marked unsteadiness, especially on movement. In these cases a total osseous labyrinthectomy may be required to control the symptoms.

Risks

1. Facial palsy.
2. Infection.
3. Perforation of the tympanic membrane.
4. Tinnitus. The loss of any residual hearing can exacerbate this symptom considerably.

Preparation

The patient is prepared as for an ossiculoplasty.

Method

1. A small endaural incision is made. A posterior tympanomeatal flap is raised. Good exposure is paramount so the ear drum should be elevated from the handle of the malleus round to the antero-inferior quadrant. The stapes and round window should be clearly visible. The incudostapedial joint is divided. The posterior meatal wall is removed with a curette in the posterosuperior quadrant to give a clear view of the pyramid and long process of the incus. The incus is removed using a pair of crocodile forceps. The stapedial tendon is cut with microscissors. The stapes is then completely removed.
2. A piece of foil is laid over the tympanomeatal flap to prevent damage from a rotating burr. A small diamond paste burr is used to widen the oval window inferiorly. The vestibule is opened gradually so that it communicates with the round window niche. The round window niche is enlarged to reveal the round window membrane. Using straight and angled cup forceps, the membranes of the inner ear are avulsed. It is important to try to avulse the membranes out of the semicircular canals.
3. Small pledgets soaked in 90% alcohol can be placed in the vestibule to destroy any remaining neuro-epithelium. They are left in place for about 10 minutes, after which the alcohol is aspirated and the vestibule irrigated with saline. A plug of fat is taken from the endaural incision and placed within the vestibule to seal the inner ear from the middle ear.
4. The foil is removed. The tympanomeatal flap is replaced and the external auditory canal packed. The endaural incision is closed with interrupted sutures.

OSSEUS LABYRINTHECTOMY

Pre-operative considerations

A three canal labyrinthectomy rarely fails to control the vertigo of acute episodes of Meniere's disease. In fact if the patient persists with episodes of acute rotatory vertigo following surgery then the diagnosis should be reconsidered or the presence of disease in the other labyrinth suspected.

A lateral canal labyrinthectomy frequently fails to control vertigo unless an ototoxic agent such as gentamicin is instilled at the time of surgery.

Risks

1. Facial palsy.
2. CSF leak.

3. Haemorrhage from a tear in the lateral venous sinus.
4. Infection which may lead to intracranial suppuration or meningitis is fortunately rare.

Preparation

The patient is prepared as for a mastoidectomy.

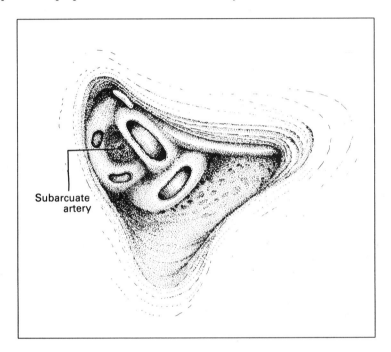

Subarcuate
artery

Figure 11.2 Fenestration of three semicircular canals (from RSE, by permission)

Method

1. A postauricular approach is made.
2. A cortical mastoidectomy is performed. The lateral semicircular canal, line of the facial nerve, dural and lateral sinuses plates are identified.
3. The three semicircular canals are drilled out, as shown in Figure 11.2. It is usual to start with a cutting burr and to open initially the lateral canal. The lateral canal is followed posteriorly. The posterior canal is now opened and traced superiorly until the superior canal is encountered. It is important to remember that the ampulla of the posterior canal usually lies deep to the facial nerve. Therefore a diamond drill is used to excise this portion of the posterior canal. Copious irrigation to cool the bone is always used close to the facial nerve. The lateral canal is next traced forwards, also using the diamond burr, maintaining a thin layer of bone covering the facial nerve. Once the canals and common crus have been excised access to the vestibule

is possible underneath the facial nerve. Care must be taken not to breach the facial canal by using a diamond drill and keeping the burr moving. The creation of 'potholes' with the drill must be avoided.

4. The membranes of the utricle and saccule are avulsed using cup forceps (Figure 11.3). In an ear free of mucosal disease the operation is now complete. However, if there is evidence of mucosal disease then the cavity may be lined with a temporalis fascia graft. Most, if not all, of any mucosal disease will have been excised during the initial cortical mastoidectomy.

5. The postauricular incision is closed in layers. The skin is closed by interrupted sutures. A pressure head bandage is applied.

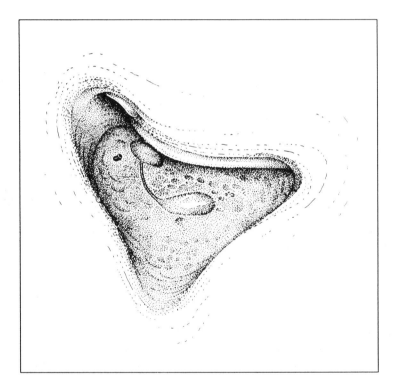

Figure 11.3 The appearance of a post-labyrynthectomy cavity showing the vestibular aqueduct and vestibule (from RSE, by permission)

Post-operative care after labyrinthectomy

1. Prophylactic penicillin is not usually required unless there has been a CSF leak. Prophylactic antibiotics should be given if there is any evidence of infected mucosa.

2. Anti-emetics should be prescribed routinely until nausea and vomiting cease.

3. The patient should be gradually mobilized. Physiotherapy exercises promote rehabilitation. The patient should not be allowed to lie in bed for days or weeks but should be encouraged to walk and take an active role in

his or her own rehabilitation. In this way permanent post-operative unsteadiness and the risk of deep vein thrombosis is minimized.
4. The pressure dressings are removed the following day and the sutures removed between 5 and 7 days.

COCHLEAR IMPLANTATION

Indications

1. Total bilateral postlingual deafness. Prelingual deafness in a child under 6 years.
2. At least one 'cochlea' should be patent on CT scan for insertion of an intracochlear electrode.
3. The best results are obtained in those patients who have been totally deaf for the shortest period of time. However, good improvement in lipreading skills and voice have been reported in patients who have been deaf for longer than 20 years prior to implantation.
4. Patients who are integrated into the deaf community present difficult psychological problems. It is possible that other deaf people, particularly those born deaf, may reject a patient after cochlear implantation and they can become social outcasts from the community in which they live. Potential patients who communicate by signing, are married to a deaf spouse or have borne deaf children should be considered most carefully. A hearing relative who is 'pushing for' the cochlear implant in an indifferent patient is virtually a surgical contra-indication.
5. Strong family or social support eases the burden of rehabilitation and mitigates in favour of a successful implant outcome.

Contra-indications

1. Born deaf, over the age of 5 years.
2. Obliteration of the cochleas or auditory cortex infarction revealed on CT scan. A single channel implant may be suitable for cases with ossified cochleas.
3. Active infection in the ear to be transplanted.
4. Unwillingness to accept the device because of cosmetic considerations.
5. Useful remaining hearing. If there is any doubt a trial of the most appropriate hearing aid should be given.
6. Ill health such that a prolonged anaesthetic carries considerable risk.
7. Physical disabilities such as blindness or paraplegia are not contra-indications to cochlear implantation.

Pre-operative considerations

1. A simple questionnaire can be sent to potential candidates and in this way certain patients, such as the born deaf, can be excluded.

2. An audiological assessment both aided and unaided should be performed to establish that a cochlear implant is likely to confer greater benefit than conventional hearing aids.
3. The patient's physical and mental suitability for surgery should be evaluated. Important background information can often be obtained from the family practitioner. In certain cases the opinion of a trained psychologist/psychiatrist can be invaluable. The expectations of these patients and their families can be unrealistic and it is important that these beliefs are thoroughly assessed.
4. Speech and lipreading skills should be assessed.
5. CT scan of temporal bones and brain.
6. Caloric tests to establish the state of vestibular function. If there is a choice between ears then the implant should be placed in the ear with the lesser caloric function. This is usually the ear with the worse hearing.
7. Care should be taken that the patient and spouse (or carer) have both the time and the motivation to follow through the rehabilitation programme.
8. There are special problems with children.
   - It must be established beyond doubt that there is no useful residual hearing.
   - The parents require considerable support.
   - The provision of an education system that allows for the special requirements of a child with a cochlear implant is most important.
9. It is vital that the infrastructure is present to rehabilitate the patient. This may consist of an audiological scientist, speech therapist and hearing therapist or psychologist. Each patient requires many hours of training in addition to the time required to educate family, employer or school. The surgeon must not be tempted to skimp on post-operative training or the patient will not achieve the full benefit of the cochlear implant.
10. The patient should be able to speak fluently the same language as the rehabilitation team. Most speech processors have been designed to cope with Indo-European languages. The effectiveness of a cochlear implant in those who speak a language that relies on the nuances of intonation is unknown.
11. The ultimate in success is probably the patient with either 100% open speech discrimination or who can use the telephone. However, any improvement from no hearing to some hearing can revolutionize a patient's life. Total failure arises when either the implant has to be removed (usually due to infection) or it is impossible to place the implant due to obliteration of the cochlea. Necrosis of the flap or breakdown of the wound usually occurs when too small a flap has been cut.
12. With careful patient selection, more than 90% of patients should benefit from surgery.

Types of implant

Multichannel intracochlear devices

There are two commonly used devices of this type:

1. The Nucleus device manufactured by the Cochlear Company of Australia is a 22 electrode device which is totally implantable. The electrodes are stimulated by an inductive link. A microphone head set is worn attached to the pinna from which a cable leads to the body-worn speech processor. The speech processor selects and codes useful speech features. The parameters which are extracted by the speech processor include the fundamental frequency, the first and second format frequencies with their relevant amplitudes and energy in three high frequency bands. The fundamental frequency is perceived as rate pitch. The formant frequencies and energy in the high frequency bands are perceived as place pitch while their amplitudes convey loudness to the patient.
2. The Ineraid manufactured by Smith Nephew Richards in the USA is a four electrode device. The electrode array is connected to the speech processor by a percutaneous stud.

Single channel devices

Several single channel devices exist which are both intracochlear and extra-cochlear devices. These devices are usually stimulated by an inductive link.

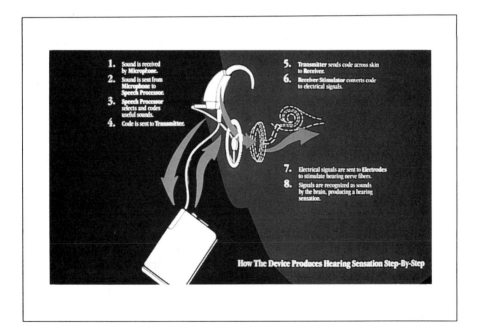

Figure 11.4 How the cochlear implant produces hearing step by step. Slide 2: Cochlear Mini 22 system slides

Risks

1. Infection of the implanted device.

2. Skin infection around the percutaneous stud is common. The stud needs careful management.
3. Damage to the percutaneous stud or the implant due to direct trauma.
4. Facial palsy.
5. Vertigo. Although the inner ear is opened at the time of implant, vertigo is rarely a problem. Often there is no labyrinth function in the operated ear. When vertigo occurs it usually settles rapidly.
6. Necrosis of the skin flaps. This should not occur provided that sufficiently large flaps are cut and that the implant is placed well away from the suture lines.
7. Involuntary facial movement. If an active electrode is in contact with the facial nerve it may stimulate that nerve. If this occurs then that electrode should be 'turned off'.
8. Inability to insert the intracochlear electrode due to obliteration of the cochlea.
9. The complications associated with cortical mastoidectomy.

Preparation

The patient should have virtually a half head shave. The patient is prepared, positioned and draped as for an extensive mastoidectomy.

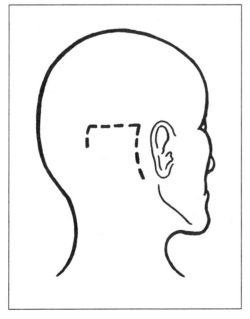

Figure 11.5 Incision line for cochlear implant

Method

1. The implantation of the Nucleus device will be described.
2. The dummy implant is placed on the skin in the approximate position for

implantation. The incision lines are drawn as an inverted U flap based inferiorly, as shown in Fig. 11.5. The incision should be approximately 1 cm from the proposed site of the implant. The flap is elevated. Rather than elevating the periosteum as a separate flap it may be excised. The temporalis muscle's inferior attachment is detached and retracted so as to reveal the bone of the skull. The external auditory canal is identified, but the meatal skin is not elevated.

3. A cortical mastoidectomy is performed. The incus and digastric ridge are found so as to identify the line of the facial nerve. A posterior tympanotomy is performed. If possible the chorda tympani is preserved. Care is taken not to damage the tympanic annulus. The round window niche and promontory are visualized through the tympanotomy. It is important not to bowl the edges of the cortical cavity (Figure 11.6).

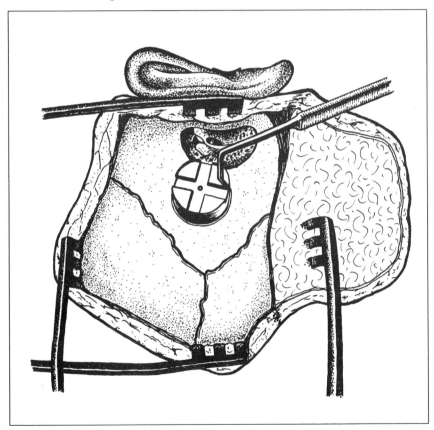

Figure 11.6 A cortical mastoidectomy with posterior tympanotomy has been performed. The site for the implant package is marked with the aid of a package. Right ear

4. A microdrill is used to create a cochleostomy (Figure 11.7). This may be done by widening the round window niche antero-inferiorly (Figure 11.8). Occasionally it is difficult to see the round window niche due to the position of the facial nerve. In this circumstance a hole can be drilled

into the cochlea just anterior to the round window. A cotton pledget is placed in the cochleostomy to prevent any bone dust entering the inner ear.

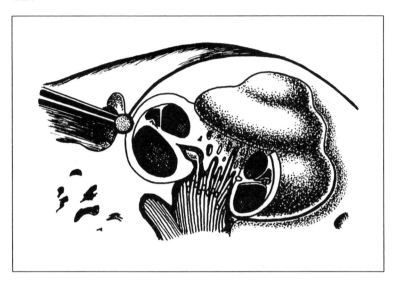

Figure 11.7   A microdrill is used to create a cochleostomy

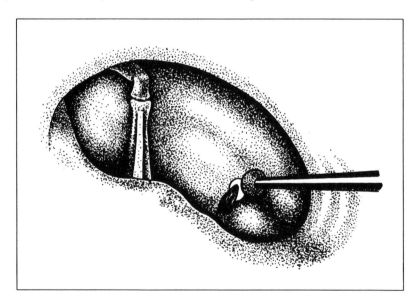

Figure 11.8   Enlarging the round window niche

5.   The site for the 'well' for implant is chosen. Using the template, a circle is drawn at the chosen site. The well is drilled out with a cutting burr and finished with the barrel-shaped diamond burr (Figure 11.9). A channel

is cut using a 2 mm thick burr between the well and the cortical mastoid cavity to take the electrode array lead (Figure 11.10).

6. Four bone anchoring sites are then drilled, two on either side of the implant, to accommodate the nylon securing suture.

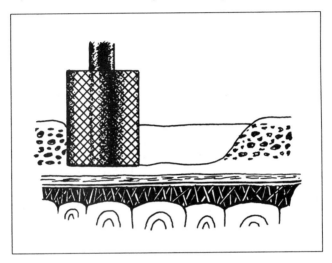

Figure 11.9 Finishing the housing for the implant

7. Before the implant is opened haemostasis is secured and the diathermy apparatus removed from the patient.
8. The implant is placed in its well and held in place with the nylon sutures. The plastic protective sheath is removed from the electrode array. The pledget is removed from the cochleostomy. The tip of the electrode array is led through the posterior tympanotomy into the cochleostomy. Using the 'forks' provided in the surgeon's implant kit, the electrode is fed into the cochlea (Figure 11.11). There are 32 electrodes, but the proximal 10 are dummies. The number of true electrodes inserted into the cochlea is recorded. The cochleostomy is plugged with fat, muscle or fascia around the electrode.
9. The proximal portion of the electrode lead is secured with either the dacron ties or, as the author favours, dental cement. The cement should not produce heat when it is mixed.
10. Haemostasis is secured, but diathermy must not be used.
11. Drains should be avoided. The wound is closed in layers. The wound may be sprayed with an antibiotic spray prior to closure.
12. A pressure head dressing is applied.

Post-operative care

1. The patient is nursed as for a mastoidectomy.
2. Prophylactic antibiotics are prescribed.
3. The pressure dressing is removed the following day.

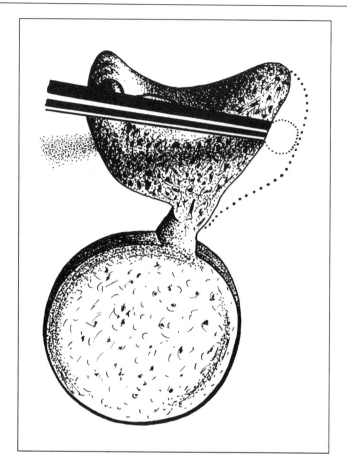

Figure 11.10   The housing completed

4. A radiograph is performed to verify that the implant is in position.
5. The position of the implant can also be verified by stimulating the electrodes after 2 or 3 days.
6. The implant is programmed about 4 weeks post-operatively.

POSTERIOR CANAL OBSTRUCTION

Indications

Severe benign paroxysmal positional vertigo which has been present for at least 12 months.

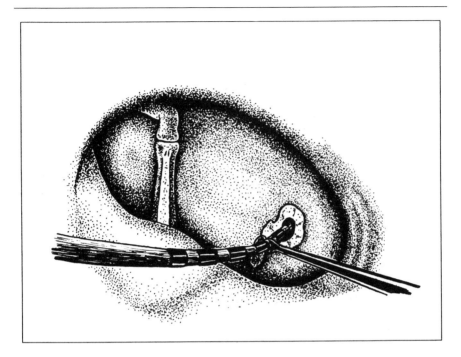

Figure 11.11   Insertion of the electrode array

Success rates

Posterior canal blocking is a new operation. Parnes described his experience of 19 cases in summer 1990 and reported an abolition of positional vertigo in all cases without any significant hearing loss. Hawthorne has performed 10 posterior canal blocking operations with complete resolution of symptoms and no significant hearing loss. One patient was left with slight unsteadiness in the dark. However, it must be borne in mind that it is too early to say if there are any long-term detrimental sequelae.

Complications

These are the same as for cortical mastoidectomy.

Pre-operative assessment

1.   Confirmation of the diagnosis by Dix Hallpike positional testing.
2.   Caloric testing.
3.   Audiometry.

Method

1.   The patient is prepared as for a cortical mastoidectomy.

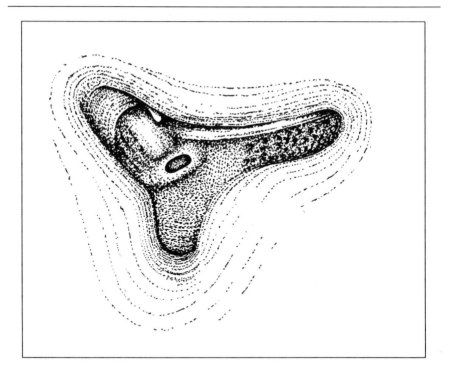

Figure 11.12   Posterior canal blocking. Right ear. Fenestration in posterior semicircular canal

2.   Via a postauricular approach, a cortical mastoidectomy is performed.
3.   The lateral semicircular canal, dural plate and lateral venous sinus are identified.
4.   The posterior semicircular canal is found at right-angles to the lateral semicircular canal between the lateral venous sinus and the lateral canal. The bone of the semicircular canals has a yellowish hue which aids in identification.
5.   The posterior semicircular canal is followed inferiorly towards the facial nerve. The ampulla lies deep to the facial nerve but it is not necessary to expose this. The posterior canal is then fenestrated. A 2 mm hole is made. Bone dust is then mixed with bone wax. Using this material, the canal is blocked. Great care is taken obstructing the canal. If possible the membranous canal is compressed without rupturing it. In this way flow through the posterior semicircular canal is blocked. A piece of temporalis fascia is laid over the fenestra.
6.   The wound is closed in layers. A pressure bandage is placed.

Post-operative care

1.   Prophylactic antibiotics and anti-emetics are prescribed.
2.   The patient is nursed and rehabilitated as for a labyrinthectomy. The patient usually has severe nausea and vomiting for about 48 hours. The patient is usually up and about after 4 days and able to return to work after 2 to 3 weeks.

Chapter 12

Surgery of the facial nerve

INTRODUCTION

The necessity to explore the facial nerve is becoming rare. The introduction of seat belt legislation and the reduction in work-related accidents has reduced the incidence of trauma to the nerve. Tumours involving the facial nerve are rare. Unfortunately, iatrogenic damage to the facial nerve still occurs, but improvement in surgical training may reduce this source.

Consequently, in order to maximize the chances of an optimal result for those few patients requiring facial nerve surgery there is an argument for one surgeon in each region to undertake this type of surgery.

EXPLORATION OF THE FACIAL NERVE

Indications

1. Immediate facial palsy as the result of trauma.
2. Delayed facial palsy following trauma where electroneuronography reveals complete denervation.
3. Immediate facial palsy following ear surgery.
4. Delayed paralysis following ear surgery may be due to a tight pack or mild contusion of the nerve. Often no surgical intervention is required as the nerve is clearly in continuity. Rarely a rapidly progressive paralysis can occur due to bleeding into the canal. Electrical studies that reveal a rapid denervation indicate the need for surgical decompression. A delayed but progressive paralysis can occur when a bone spicule is driven into the nerve. A poor outcome can result from subsequent intra-neural fibrosis.
5. Occasionally a patient may be referred late. The optimal time for nerve exploration may have passed. If referral is within 8 weeks and the paralysis is complete then exploration should be performed, especially if the palsy was immediate in onset or there is evidence of complete degeneration on electrical testing. After 8 weeks it is worth waiting and performing EMG to identify any polyphasic action potentials indicating reinervation. If there is no evidence of recovery after 4 months then the nerve should be explored.

After 1 year exploration carries little advantage.
6. Facial nerve neuroma. Tumours involving the facial nerve.
7. Selective neurectomy for hemifacial spasm or blepharospasm.

Pre-operative considerations

1. It is difficult to generalize as to the effectiveness of facial nerve surgery because the diagnosis and the length of time that any facial palsy has been present influences the result.
2. For an iatrogenic facial palsy the earlier the exploration and grafting are performed the better the result.
3. Graft anastomoses should not be under tension. Twin cable grafts appear to confer a slight advantage over a single cable graft.
4. Decompression of the neuropraxic nerve will result in full recovery. The degenerated nerve in continuity will recover provided there is no obstruction such as intra-neural fibrosis or a bone spicule.
5. Recovery of the degenerated nerve will take between 6 and 18 months.
6. In the totally sectioned nerve, nerve grafting gives the best results.
7. Nearly all cases with a facial nerve graft have some return of facial symmetry with eye closure.

Risks

1. Additional damage to the facial nerve.
2. Conductive deafness.
3. Sensorineural deafness.
4. Vertigo.
5. CSF leak, especially following the middle fossa approach to the internal auditory meatus.
6. Extradural haematoma (following the middle fossa approach).
7. Troublesome intra-operative haemorrhage can occur from the venous and arterial structures that traverse the foramen spinosum. These may be damaged during the middle fossa approach.
8. Facial paralysis leads to exposure of the cornea. Corneal damage can occur both at the time of surgery or in the post-operative period.

EXPOSURE OF THE FACIAL NERVE IN THE FACE

This is described under superficial parotidectomy in Chapter 13. The facial nerve should be identified in an area of normal anatomy. The nerve may be found where it exits the styloid foramen; however, it is important to be able to identify the peripheral branches.
1. The parotid gland does not typically extend above the zygomatic arch. The two superior branches of the facial nerve are in contact with the periosteum and fascia over the zygomatic arch.
2. Buccal branches can be identified because of their constant relationship to the parotid duct. Such branches run parallel to the duct both above and below the duct.

3. The marginal mandibular branch can be safely identified. The retromandibular vein is identified about 2 cm below the angle of the jaw. The vein is then carefully followed superiorly. The marginal mandibular branch of the facial is encountered where it crosses superficial to the vein.
4. The use of a facial nerve stimulator and magnification are invaluable to the surgeon in rapidly identifying the fine peripheral branches of the facial nerve.

EXPOSURE OF THE TYMPANOMASTOID SEGMENT OF THE FACIAL NERVE

The approach to the horizontal segment depends very much on the presence or absence of hearing loss. In the patient with normal hearing and an intact ossicular chain an approach to the horizontal segment via the mastoid is fraught with difficulties. It is extremely difficult to remove bone from the canal of the nerve without touching the ossicular chain. The horizontal portion of the nerve can be approached with much less risk to hearing via the middle fossa.

Method

1. A cortical mastoidectomy is performed via a postauricular approach (see Chapter 10).
2. It is important to identify the following landmarks: the dural plate, the incus, the sigmoid sinus, the digastric ridge and the lateral semicircular canal.
3. The line of the facial nerve is identified. The digastric ridge is followed forward to encounter the facial nerve (Figure 12.1). The bone of the mastoid tip is drilled away to expose the tough periosteum that covers the nerve. As it is followed forward the periosteum funnels into the stylomastoid foramen. A large diamond burr cooled with copious irrigation is used to expose the nerve sheath.

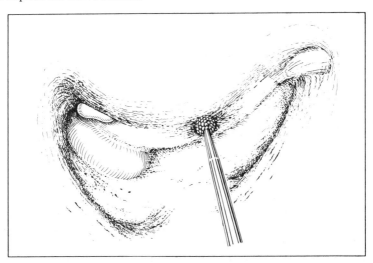

Figure 12.1 Skeletonization of the facial nerve in a mastoid segment using the landmarks of the short process of the incus, lateral semicircular canal, and digastric ridge (from RSE, by permission)

4. A posterior tympanotomy is performed. In this way the entire descending portion of the facial nerve can be exposed without disturbing the external auditory canal and the tympanic membrane (Figure 12.2).

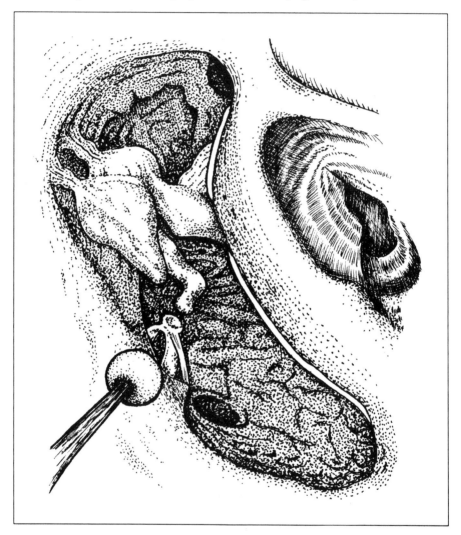

Figure 12.2 A posterior tympanotomy to reveal the facial nerve. Note that the incudostapedial joint has been disarticulated in order to prevent sensorineural deafness

5. The horizontal portion can be safely approached via the mastoid when the patient has a 'dead ear'. After exposing the descending portion of the nerve a posterosuperior tympanomeatal flap is raised. The outer attic wall is removed with a drill via the meatus to expose the ossicular heads. The tympanomeatal flap is protected with an aluminium foil sheet from the rotating burr. Care is taken not to breach the posterior meatal wall. The incus and head of the malleus are removed. Using a diamond paste drill,

the bone over the horizontal facial canal is thinned. The bone of the facial canal is carefully removed with a raspatory.

6. After repair of the nerve a temporalis fascia graft and a small piece of conchal cartilage are harvested. The conchal cartilage is shaped to fit the attic defect. The temporalis fascia is 'underlaid' beneath the tympanomeatal flap and over the conchal cartilage repair. A dressing is placed in the external auditory canal and the post-auricular wound closed.

7. An alternative to the above technique is to create a radical mastoid cavity. The skin of the external auditory canal is completely excised. The residual cuff of the external auditory canal skin is everted and the ear canal closed. The malleus, incus and tympanic membrane are excised. The mucosa of the middle ear cleft is removed. The bony auditory tube is widened by removing bone from all round the orifice except the medial aspect where the internal carotid artery runs. The auditory tube is blocked with muscle and bone wax. Once the nerve has been repaired the cavity is packed with fat from the subcutaneous layer of the abdomen. The temporalis muscle is mobilized and swung down into the mastoid defect and sutured in place. Finally, the postauricular wound is closed.

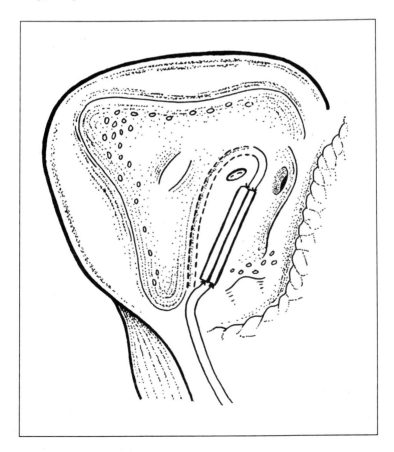

Figure 12.3 A twin cabled graft of the facial nerve re-routed across the promontory between the horizontal segment and the stylomastoid foramen

The main advantage of the radical cavity is that the facial nerve may be mobilized and re-routed across the cavity from the geniculate ganglion to the stylomastoid foramen (Figure 12.3). In this technique an end-to-end nerve anastomosis may be possible rather than having to insert a graft.

MIDDLE FOSSA APPROACH

The horizontal, labyrinthine and internal meatal portions of the facial nerve may be approached by this route. Pre-operative investigations should include CT scanning of the petrous temporal bone, audiometry, caloric testing and any electrophysiological tests of facial nerve function that are appropriate.

Preparation

The temporal region is shaved. The patient, under general anaesthesia with endotracheal intubation, is positioned in a supine position with the head rotated to one side. The surgeon sits at the head of the table.

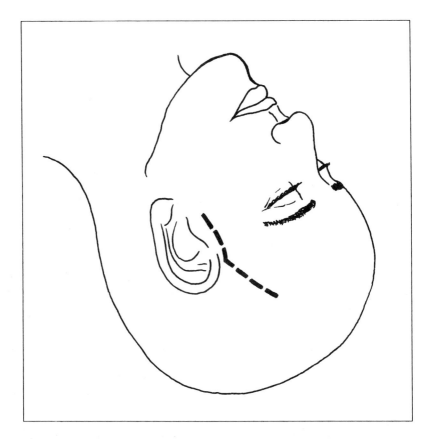

Figure 12.4   Incision for the middle fossa approach to the internal auditory meatus

Method

1. The incision extends superiorly from the tragus to the superior margin of the temporalis muscle (Figure 12.4). The incision is deepened to the temporalis muscle. The temporalis fascia is exposed by blunt dissection and the wound held open with self-retaining retractors.
2. An inferiorly based temporalis flap is cut up to the superior attachment of the muscle. The flap is about 2 cm wide. This flap is reflected inferiorly. The temporalis muscle remaining is retracted to expose the skull (Figure 12.5).

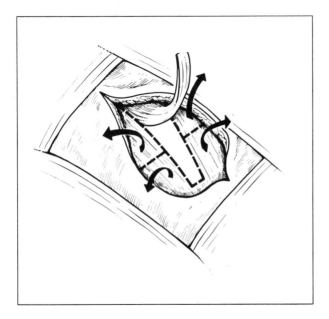

Figure 12.5   The temporalis muscle flap is cut. Left ear (from RSE, by permission)

3. A 3 cm × 2 cm craniotomy flap is cut using a 2 mm burr. The bone flap is centred over the root of the zygoma (Figure 12.6). The lower border of the bone flap is about 1 cm above the zygoma. The inferior border of the craniotomy is enlarged using bone rongeurs. This gives a good view of the petrosquamous attachment of the dura. The dura is lifted with a dural hook and nicked with a knife to release the CSF.
4. The temporal lobe dura is gradually elevated from the bone of the middle cranial fossa (Figure 12.7). Bipolar diathermy is used to coagulate veins found along the base of the middle cranial fossa. It is unnecessary to expose the foramen spinosum. The arcuate eminence and bone over the internal auditory canal is exposed. Elevation anteriorly is stopped after exposure of the facial hiatus. A self-retaining dura retractor with a Cushing retractor is placed in the wound.
5. With the aid of magnification, a diamond paste burr is used to remove the bone over the arcuate eminence. The compact yellowish bone of the superior semicircular canal is exposed just a little anterior to the arcuate

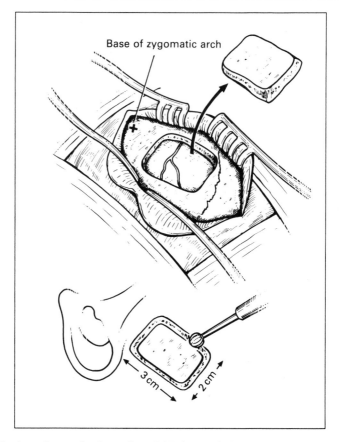

Figure 12.6 A craniotomy flap is cut (from RSE, by permission)

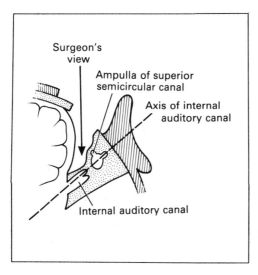

Figure 12.7 Coronal view of the approach to the internal auditory canal (from RSE, by permission)

eminence. The superior semicircular canal is 'blue lined' to identify it clearly. The internal auditory canal is found in a line about 60° anterior to the semicircular canal (Figure 12.8). Bone is removed in a 60° sector anterior to the semicircular canal. Thus the 'blue' of the meatal fundus is exposed. The meatal fundus is exposed and the vertical crest identified. This allows the facial nerve to be found.

6. The meatal roof is carefully removed using a diamond burr. The facial nerve is exposed in the labyrinthine segment.

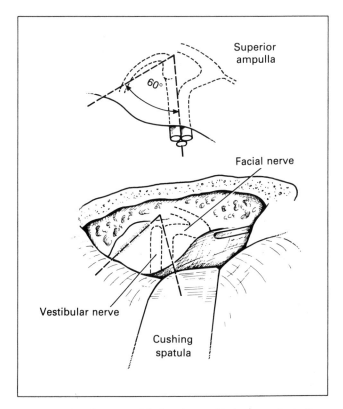

Figure 12.8 The internal auditory canal is found at a 60 degree angle to the superior semicircular canal. Left ear (from RSE, by permission)

7. The roof of the middle ear is very carefully opened. Great care must be taken not to damage the ossicles. The surgeon may wish to consider dislocating the incudostapedial joint via a tympanotomy before commencing the middle fossa approach. After exposure of the geniculate ganglion the facial nerve may be followed into the horizontal segment.

8. Once the nerve has been repaired a free muscle graft is placed in the widened internal auditory canal. The roof of the middle ear is closed by placing a piece of the craniotomy bone flap or a piece of conchal cartilage over the defect. The inferiorly based muscle pedicle is laid into the defect and the dural retractors removed.

9.   The bone flap is replaced. The temporalis muscle is sutured over the defect. A low pressure suction drain is placed in the anterior portion of the wound. The wound is closed with interrupted sutures and the drain secured to the skin.

Donor sites of nerve grafts

1.   Greater auricular nerve. This is a convenient nerve to harvest for grafting. It has the major advantage of branching in such a fashion that it is a good graft for repairing the facial nerve in the face. However, the main trunk is a little short. Four centimetres of graft is usually the maximum length available. The nerve can be found in the lower limb of the conventional parotidectomy incision where it crosses the sternomastoid muscle.
2.   Lateral cutaneous nerve of the thigh (Figure 12.9). This has the advantage of giving a potential donor length of up to 10 cm. When this nerve is harvested it leaves the patient with a numb area on the lateral aspect of the thigh. The nerve is found by first identifying the inguinal ligament. The nerve is found about 2 cm medial to the anterior superior iliac spine and about 2 cm inferior to the ligament.
3.   Sural nerve. The sural nerve supplies sensation to the lateral border of the foot. When taken as a donor nerve it can provide considerable length in excess of 10 cm. However, anaesthesia of the lateral border of the foot can lead to ulceration of the skin especially due to ill-fitting shoes. The nerve can be found where it passes posterior and inferior to the lateral malleolus.

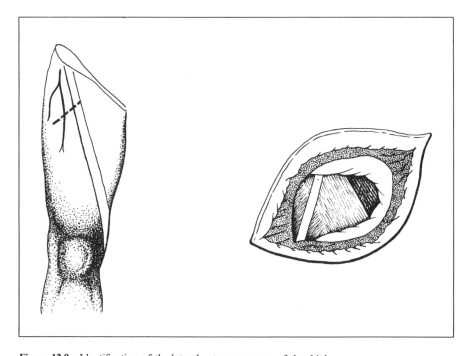

Figure 12.9   Identification of the lateral cutaneous nerve of the thigh

Techniques of nerve repair

Several techniques of nerve repair have been described and each has its exponents. However, all techniques have two factors in common:

- The ends of the nerve should be cleanly cut so that the fascicles are exposed and there is minimal trauma.
- The anastomosis should not be under tension.

Attempting to perform an anastomosis in the cerebellopontine angle is difficult. Firstly, the stump has no significant sheath and is soft. Secondly, the pulsation of the CSF means that the stump is usually waving around and difficult to hold atraumatically. The graft is also floating in the CSF. The surgeon is operating in a 'deep hole' hampered by the close proximity of vessels and brain stem. Using 9/0 monofilament nylon, the surgeon is usually pleased if he or she can get one or two stitches placed to bring the ends into apposition.

Within the temporal bone the surgeon can usually drill a gutter in which to place the nerve. At its simplest, the two ends of nerve may be laid end to end and wrapped in fascia, or a processed material such as Cargile. Other surgeons use a tissue glue such as fibrin glue or a mixture of cryoprecipitate and thrombin.

If the anastomosis may be pulled apart by muscle movement such as in the face then suture should be used. The fascicles can be dissected out and a single 10/0 suture used to anastomose each individual fascicle. The authors favour suturing the epineurium with 9/0 monofilament material. This gives a neat anastomosis and an acceptable result with about four or five stitches.

Twin cable grafts have been shown in animal research to give superior results over single cable grafts. Furthermore, grafts of less than 1 cm long give poorer results than when the graft is longer than 1 cm.

Post-operative care

1. If the cranial cavity has been opened then the patients have initially quarter-hourly neurological observations, including pulse, blood pressure, pupillary responses and conscious level. The temperature should be taken four-hourly. As soon as the patient has regained full consciousness he or she should be nursed sitting up and the frequency of the nursing observations may be reduced.
2. If the cranial cavity has been opened the patient should be forbidden from nose blowing lest air is forced through the ear via the craniotomy into the cranial cavity.
3. Prophylactic penicillin should be prescribed.
4. The eye will require protection until the nerve graft has 'taken'. This may be by a temporary tarsorrhaphy or botulinum toxin may be injected into the levator palpebrae superiores. The tarsorrhaphy has the advantage that the patient can still see out of the eye as the lid is not completely closed. A tarsorrhaphy can cause problems with entropion and in growing of the eyelashes even after it has been undone. This lash problem does not occur with botulinum toxin but the patient cannot see because of the complete ptosis which has been induced.

Chapter 13

Salivary gland surgery

SURGERY FOR A RANULA

Indications

A ranula is a retention cyst in the anterior floor of the mouth which arises from obstruction to the duct of a lingual salivary gland. If there is difficulty with swallowing or speech due to reduced tongue movement then surgical removal is indicated. Patients often wish the ranula removed for cosmetic reasons.

Specimen

The cyst plus the associated salivary gland should be excised.

Pre-operative considerations

A ranula should be distinguished from a cystic hygroma involving the floor of the mouth.

Preparation

General anaesthesia through a pernasal endotracheal tube with a protective throat pack inserted is preferable. Local infiltration anaesthesia can be used for this operation (lignocaine 2%, 1:200 000 adrenaline). The patient is supine with the head supported on a head ring.

Risks

1.   Haematoma in the floor of the mouth.

2. Submandibular duct obstruction.
3. Lingual nerve damage.
4. Recurrence of the ranula.

Method

1. A Doyen gag is inserted and a stout tongue stay suture placed through the mid-line raphe of the anterior tongue.
2. The tip of the tongue is elevated to reveal and place on the stretch the floor of mouth ranula. A pair of forceps grasps the anterior tip of the ranula and distracts the cyst inferiorly.
3. Scalpel and then fine dissecting scissors are used to develop the plane of dissection between the cyst and the tongue substance. Gauze or pledget dissection can be helpful. It is important not to stray from the correct plane.
4. Dissection into the cyst increases the risk of recurrence, whereas dissection into the tongue risks troublesome haemorrhage. At the most posterior part of the dissection the lingual nerve and the submandibular duct are at risk.
5. Mucosa can be opposed with absorbable sutures to close the wound if necessary, but it is important to avoid catching or damaging the submandibular duct.

Post-operative care

The patient should be observed post-operatively to ensure that an expanding haematoma of the floor of the mouth does not occur. A normal to soft diet is usually possible the day following surgery.

SUBMANDIBULAR GLAND EXCISION

Indications

1. Recurrent enlargement of the gland caused by duct obstruction, which may be caused by stones (common), radiotherapy or surgery to the floor of mouth.
2. Suspected malignancy.
3. As part of another procedure, such as radical neck dissection.

Specimen

Submandibular gland.

Pre-operative considerations

The mandibular branch of the facial nerve is at risk. This nerve runs in the fascia deep to platysma, usually about 2 cm below the horizontal ramus of the mandible. In the elderly the nerve may have a particularly low course. Figure 13.1 shows the course of this nerve and related anatomy. The skin incision should avoid this nerve. The lingual nerve and hypoglossal nerve are also at risk in the deep part of the dissection.

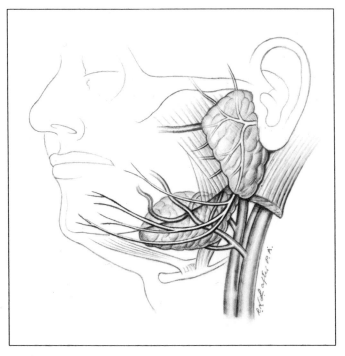

Figure 13.1   Relationship of the inferior branches of the facial nerve to the submandibular gland (from RSN, by permission)

Risks

1. Haematoma as a result of failure to drain the wound or very early removal of the drain.
2. Paralysis of the mandibular division of the facial nerve results in a droop at the corner of the mouth which may never recover.
3. Tongue anaesthesia from lingual nerve damage.
4. Hypoglossal nerve damage.

Preparation

General anaesthesia through a nasal or oral endotracheal tube. The patient is supine with a sandbag under the shoulders to extend the neck, a headring to support the head and the point of chin rotated to the opposite side from the surgery.

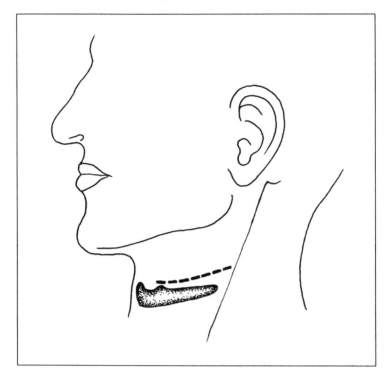

Figure 13.2   Incision for exposure of the submandibular gland

Method

1. A horizontal skin crease incision two finger breadths below the angle of the mandible at the level of the hyoid bone is deepened through platysma and cervical fascia on to the lower margin of the gland. Figure 13.2 shows the siting of the incision.
2. The fascial cuff is elevated superiorly, exposing the gland and protecting the mandibular branch of the nerve.
3. The gland grasped in forceps is dissected deep to its capsule:
   - Postero-inferiorly – the facial artery and common facial vein require ligation and division, the posterior belly of digastric is identified and the hypoglossal nerve may be identified lying on hyoglossus deep to digastric.
   - Superiorly – facial artery and vein may require ligation and division a second time.
   - Anteriorly – the superficial lobe of the gland is dissected posteriorly and freed from the posterior margin of the mylohyoid muscle.
4. The mylohyoid muscle is retracted forward by a small blunt retractor and the gland pulled inferiorly (Figure 13.3). This demonstrates the lingual nerve which is then separated from the gland and duct. The submandibular duct is ligated as far anterior as is possible and the gland removed.

5.   A suction drain is inserted and the wound closed in two layers with absorbable sutures to platysma and non-absorbable sutures or clips to skin.

Post-operative care

The drain is removed when there is a minimum of drainage, usually after 24 to 48 hours.

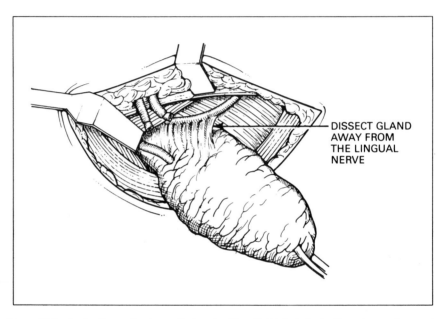

DISSECT GLAND
AWAY FROM
THE LINGUAL
NERVE

Figure 13.3   As the dissected submandibular gland is pulled inferiorly the lingual nerve frequently comes into view (from OGS, by permission)

SUPERFICIAL PAROTIDECTOMY

Indications

1.   A swelling in the parotid region which is suspected of being neoplastic.
2.   Chronic sialadenitis and chronic suppurative parotitis (rare).
3.   As part of a total parotidectomy or infratemporal resection.

Specimen

Superficial lobe of the parotid gland.

Pre-operative considerations

The facial nerve is at risk. The patient should be aware of the potential consequences of facial nerve paralysis in terms of facial appearance and eye closure. Fine needle aspiration biopsy is useful to enable the surgeon to give the patient pre-operative prognostic information.

Risks

1. Haematoma as a result of failure to drain the wound or very early removal of the drain.
2. Facial nerve paralysis. Depending on the specific nature of the surgery, a temporary or partial facial palsy may occur.
3. Anaesthesia over the elevated skin flap nearly always occurs.
4. Frey's (auriculotemporal) syndrome is gustatory sweating and occurs in a high proportion of patients if deliberately asked for. This condition tends to resolve spontaneously and only a small percentage of patients have a persistent problem.

Preparation

General anaesthesia through a nasal or oral endotracheal tube. Neuromuscular blocking agents should be avoided to allow the facial nerve to be stimulated intra-operatively. The patient is supine on the table, neck extended, point of chin rotated to the opposite side with the corner of mouth and ipsilateral eye exposed. Cotton wool in the external meatus helps to prevent blood clot forming in the external meatus as this can be uncomfortable post-operatively. Controlled hypotension improves the surgical field.

Method

1. Figure 13.4 shows the incision for superficial parotidectomy. It commences in the skin crease anterior to the pinna, curves behind the ear lobe to the tip of the mastoid bone and then runs forward in a skin crease at the level of the hyoid bone.
2. The incision is deepened in the upper part to the fascial layer superficial to the parotid gland and in the lower part through the platysma muscle. The greater auricular nerve (or its terminal branches) is divided in the lower part of the incision at the anterior border of the sternomastoid.
3. A flap with skin and subcutaneous tissue is elevated from the parotid gland until the anterior, inferior and superior borders of the superficial lobe are visible. Care has to be taken not to damage branches of the facial nerve as they exit from the borders of the gland – particularly at risk are the branches to the eye.
4. The posterior margin of the superficial lobe is freed from the upper part of the sternomastoid muscle. A stay suture is placed in the ear lobe and the pinna retracted posterosuperiorly.

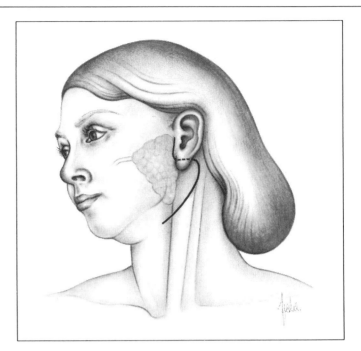

Figure 13.4   Incision for parotidectomy (from RSN, by permission)

5. A wide tunnel (3–4 cm) is created anterior to the external auditory meatus. Dissection is at the level of the perichondrium. Retraction of the sternomastoid postero-inferiorly allows identification of the underlying posterior belly of digastric which helps in the identification of the nerve.

6. The facial nerve can be identified by a number of landmarks:
    *   The nerve is 1 cm medial and 1 cm inferior to the tragal cartilage pointer.
    *   The nerve bisects the angle formed by the posterior belly of digastric and tympanomastoid bone.
    *   The nerve issues at the distal part of the tympanomastoid suture.

7. Figure 13.5 shows the tunnel to identify the nerve. Once the facial nerve is identified (a nerve stimulator facilitates this) artery clip forceps are opened along the line of the nerve. Superficial parotid gland is dissected from the branches of the facial nerve by insinuating and opening the artery clip along the line of the nerve, testing the tissue under tension with the nerve stimulator and then dividing the tissue away from the nerve. This is shown in Figure 13.6. Dissection proceeds to the limits of the gland.

8. There is a prominent vein which runs from the inferior pole of the gland. It is preferable not to divide this vein until late in the procedure as this prevents venous congestion within the gland.

9. The facial nerve can also be identified at the anterior margin of the gland close to the parotid duct. The buccal branch can be found approximately 5 mm superior to the duct. It is possible to follow the nerve to its main trunk from this point.

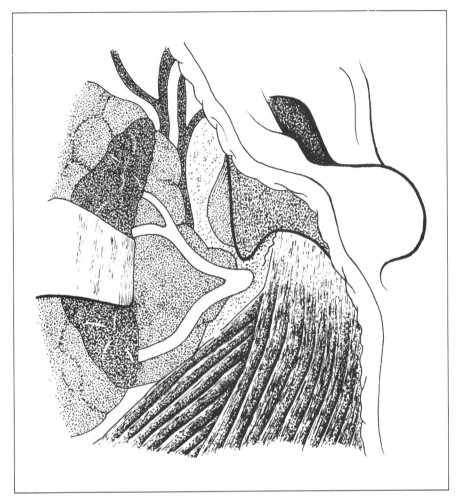

Figure 13.5 Identification of the facial nerve just anterior to the posterior belly of digastric. The tragal pointer can also be seen

10. Methods have been described to identify and follow backwards the mandibular nerve and the branches to the eyes. Although these methods have their expert exponents the authors suggest that these methods are not for the inexperienced. Once the facial nerve is dissected free it is a simple matter to remove the superficial lobe of the parotid.

11. At the conclusion of the surgery it is important to check the integrity of the facial nerve with a stimulator. If there is a loss of facial muscle stimulation one should look for disconnection of the stimulator, a haematoma of the nerve or division of the nerve. A haematoma should be incised with a sickle knife. Re-anastomosis or cable grafting will be required in cases of facial nerve division.

12. When haemostasis is secure (hypotension reversed) a suction drain is inserted and the wound closed in two layers with absorbable sutures to

platysma and non-absorbable sutures or clips to skin. The suture line should be airtight.

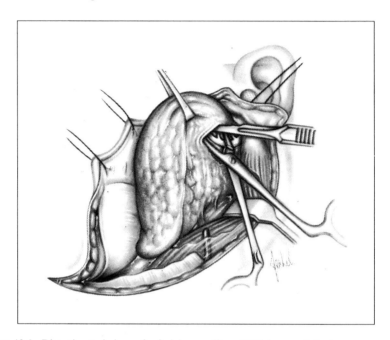

Figure 13.6   Dissection technique of a facial nerve (from RSN, by permission)

Post-operative care

The integrity of the facial nerve should be noted as soon as the patient awakes from the anaesthetic to give a baseline for subsequent management. A partial weakness of the facial musculature is very common in a thoroughly performed superficial parotidectomy. A normal diet and full mobilization would be expected the day following surgery. The vacuum drain is removed after 24–48 hours when the aspirate is less than 10 ml in the preceding 24 hours. Discharge from hospital is generally 1 to 2 days after removal of the drain.

Chapter 14

Principles of nasal and sinus surgery

INTRODUCTION

Vision

Good illumination is mandatory in the performance of nasal and paranasal sinus surgery. A headlight is usually adequate in most instances, although in certain circumstances the endoscopic nasal telescope is superior. In some situations, such as surgery of the pterygopalatine fossa, an operating microscope is useful and in this case a 300 mm lens is the ideal objective lens. If nasal hairs obstruct vision into the nasal cavity they should be cut. Light can be provided directly to the site of surgery via a fibre-optic system attached to operating instruments such as a Killian's speculum.

Suction

Adequate suction is always required. The Zoellner sucker can be appropriate for intra-nasal surgery, though often a wider bore sucker may be appropriate for paranasal sinus work. Bipolar diathermy can be helpful, although applying a unipolar diathermy to the shaft of a Zoellner sucker can be a useful technique of controlling bleeding in paranasal sinus surgery. Figure 14.1 shows the Zoellner sucker sheathed with a size 10 nasogastric tube to protect from accidental diathermy burns.

Haemostasis

1. Good haemostasis within nasal and paranasal sinus surgery is essential. For intranasal surgery the mucosal lining should be prepared prior to transfer to the operating room. This can be performed satisfactorily with xylometazoline (Otrivine) or its long-acting derivative oxymetazoline (Afrazine). In some centres a lignocaine and adrenaline or a cocaine mixture may be used to vasoconstrict the nasal lining, but these drugs carry greater systemic complications than Otrivine or its derivatives.
2. The subperiosteal and subperichondrial layer of the septum is infiltrated with a vasoconstrictive solution such as 1:200 000 adrenaline prior to septal surgery to develop the correct blood-free plane.

3. Many surgeons combine a local anaesthetic drug with vasoconstrictive solutions to prepare the nose for surgery. The solutions used vary in concentration between surgeons from lignocaine 2%, 1:80 000 adrenaline to lignocaine 0.5%, 1:200 000 adrenaline. Other surgeons use octapressin combined with felypressin. It is important for the surgeon to liaise with the anaesthetist over the types and dosages of drugs used to prepare the nose. Many anaesthetists prophylactically 'beta block' their anaesthetized patients to counteract the local anaesthetic ministrations of the surgeon. It is always important to give the local anaesthetic/vasoconstrictive agent time to work prior to performing surgery.

4. The anaesthetist may help with hypotensive anaesthetic techniques and raising the head of the table may help in the creation of a 'dry' surgical field.

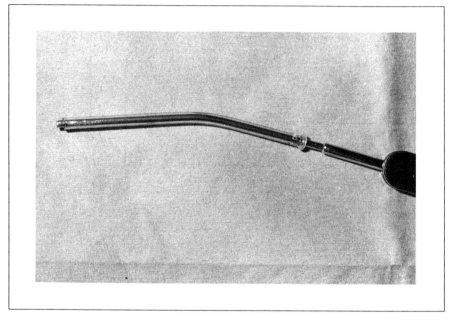

Figure 14.1   Zoellner sucker with sheath (size 10 French Gauge), for use with unipolar diathermy.

Instrumentation

1. It is important to differentiate between soft tissue and punch forceps for nasal and paranasal sinus surgery. Forceps such as the Tilly Henckel are for soft tissue removal.

2. When removing bone it is important that the punch forceps remove the bone without any tearing action. A tearing action can result in a fracture line which within the nose may extend to damage the cribriform plate or within the face of the maxilla may extend to damage the infraorbital nerve. Punch forceps, such as the Luc's or Irwin Moore, are good for nibbling thin pieces of bone, while the heavier punch forceps, such as the Jansen Middleton punch forceps, are for removing septal bone. The Ferris Smith

or Kerison punch forceps are ideal for removal of bone from the anterior face of the maxilla and maxillary process of the frontal bone.

3. A drill and rotating burr can often be of use to remove bone during paranasal sinus surgery. This instrument is also very useful to smooth rough edges within a surgically created paranasal sinus cavity. Rough edges will initially snag any packing and will subsequently be areas in which granulation tissue forms.

4. A set of Freer knives, elevators or instruments of a similar nature are required to elevate mucoperichondrial/mucoperiosteal flaps, particularly from the nasal septum. It is important that 'flaps' are raised in the subperichondrial planes as this ensures that the vital blood supply which runs in the perichondrial layer is preserved. The nature of the blood supply to the nasal septal mucosa is shown in Figure 14.2. Freer's elevator and knives are good examples of instruments whose tips are well designed to preserve the mucoperichondrial layers.

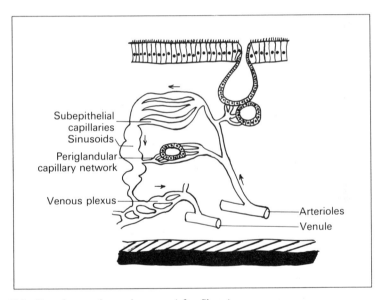

Figure 14.2   Vascular supply nasal mucosa (after Slome)

Elevation of nasal septal flaps

The elevation of a nasal septal mucoperichondrial/mucoperiosteal flap requires that the correct plane is first identified. A scalpel blade is used to cut down on to the septal cartilage and then the plane is identified. A pair of fine, curved sharp pointed dissecting scissors or the scraping action of a scalpel can be used to demonstrate the plane. Elevation of the flap should be on a broad front – tunnelling can result in tears of the flap. To free a flap from the apex of either a vertical or horizontal spur by direct dissection will result generally in a tear of the flap. It is better to dissect the flap from the concave side of the spur and to excise the piece of cartilage from the mucosa at the apex.

OPERATIVE PLANNING FOR NASAL TUMOUR SURGERY

When planning surgery within the paranasal sinuses one should consider the pathology of the lesion and if necessary organize CT scans, MRI scans or angiography to determine the precise site and vascularity of the tumour. MRI has the added advantage of being able to distinguish tumour from associated inflammatory changes in the mucosa. If there is considerable blood supply to the tumour then one can either ligate the feeding blood vessels or perform embolization prior to the surgery.

It is important to consider whether the tumour encroaches on intra-cranial, orbital or dental structures so that, if appropriate, the neurosurgeon, ophthalmic surgeon or oral surgeon can be involved in the operative management from the outset.

Risks of nasal and paranasal sinus surgery

When considering the risks of nasal and paranasal sinus surgery one should consider the structures, nerve supplies and blood supplies which are at risk from the surgical procedure.

1.   Dental damage

The nerve and blood supply to the upper dentition can be damaged during septal surgery (particularly work around the anterior nasal spine) and during surgery to the maxillary sinus. Most commonly this occurs with sublabial approaches to the maxillary sinus, but can occasionally follow intra-nasal antrostomy.

2.   Orbital problems

Surgery around the orbit can cause disruption to the orbital contents. This may result in minimal diplopia following surgery such as ligature of the anterior ethmoidal artery or may be more severe if the entire medial wall of the orbit is removed. Damage to the optic nerve and consequent blindness is a potential risk of surgery to the posterior ethmoidal air cells. A post-operative intra-orbital haematoma may compromise the blood supply to the optic nerve which may result in blindness if it is not identified, vision monitored and appropriate treatment instituted. Obstruction to the nasolacrimal duct during paranasal sinus surgery may result in epiphora. It is interesting, however, how seldom epiphora occurs, even in patients who have nasal packs.

3.   Cutaneous anaesthesia

Cutaneous nerve supplies can be affected during many rhinological and paranasal sinus operations. The infra-orbital nerve is at risk during sublabial procedures and is inevitably cut during the performance of a maxillectomy (Weber Ferguson) incision. Supraorbital and supratrochlear nerves supplying sensation to the forehead can be damaged during eyebrow incisions and approaches to the frontal ethmoidal complex. Cutaneous anaesthesia almost always occurs over the bridge and tip of the nose following elevation of the skin during a rhinoplasty.

4.   Cosmesis

The cosmetic results of nasal and paranasal sinus surgery will depend on the procedure performed. It is important to realize that a very slight supratip depression is common following septal surgery. The design of the facial incisions as approaches to the paranasal sinuses are usually cosmetically acceptable. The exact incisions will be discussed later. Figure 14.3 demonstrates the common facial incisions for approaches to the paranasal sinuses.

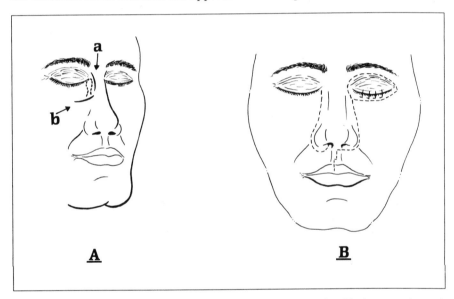

Figure 14.3(A) The superior incision is used to approach the ethmoid sinus complex and sphenoid sinus (a). The lower incision gives an approach to both the ethmoid air cell system and the maxillary antrum (b). **(B)** The right hand-sided incision for lateral rhinotomy, the left-hand incision for maxillectomy with and without preservation of orbital contents

APPROACHES TO THE PARANASAL SINUSES AND POST-NASAL SPACE

One can approach pathology within the nose, paranasal sinuses and post-nasal space through a number of routes.

1.   Pernasal

One can approach the paranasal sinuses and post-nasal space through the nose, either aided by a headlight or with the use of an endoscope.

2.   Sublabial

The sublabial route can be taken to approach the maxillary and ethmoidal air cells, but there is some limitation in access to the frontal ethmoidal complex. Neurosurgeons often use a sublabial transeptal approach to the pituitary fossa. Figure 14.4 shows a bilateral sublabial approach with facial degloving to both maxillary sinuses and the nasal cavity.

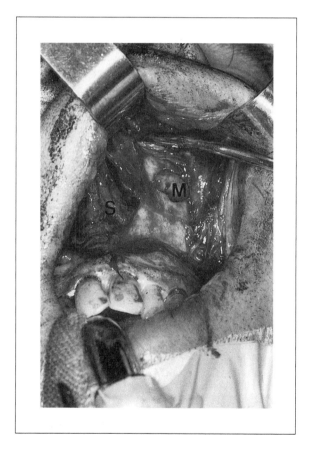

Figure 14.4 This shows a bilateral sublabial facial degloving approach. The retraction on the lip can be altered to expose different parts of both maxillary sinuses and the nasal cavity. S marks the nasal septum while M shows a fenestration into the left maxillary sinus.

3.   Through the mouth

It is possible to approach the post-nasal space through the mouth. At its simplest a retractor is used to pull the soft palate forwards and get an improved view into the post-nasal space. Alternatively, soft rubber catheters are passed through each side of the nose and used as retractors of the soft palate.

4. Transpalatal

If access to the post-nasal space is inadequate with simple retraction then a transpalatal approach can be used. Figure 14.5 shows some of the incisions which can be used in a transpalatal approach to the post-nasal space. Where the mucosa of the entire hard palate is to be elevated, the incision should be medial to the teeth and lateral to the greater palatine foramina. If only a short flap of hard palate mucosa is to be elevated then the incision should be medial to both maxillary tuberosities and the greater palatine foramina, thus ensuring adequate blood supply to both hard and soft palate, soft tissues.

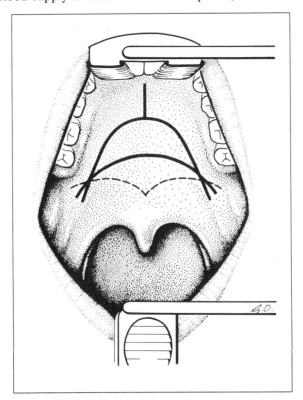

Figure 14.5   Transpalatal approach incision lines (from RSN, by permission)

Good access to the post-nasal space alone can be obtained through an incision placed immediately anterior to the posterior margin of the hard palate. This incision is deepened through mucosa and periosteum down to bone. Closure at the end of the procedure is facilitated by undermining the anterior flap at the time of the initial incision. The posterior flap is then elevated and dissected free from the posterior surface of the hard palate. Figure 14.6 shows the exposure which can be obtained through a transpalatal approach. If the tumour extends into the nasal cavity or that access is inadequate it is possible to extend the bony opening anteriorly using punch forceps to the floor of the nose. The wound is closed in one layer with absorbable sutures, such as vicryl or dexon.

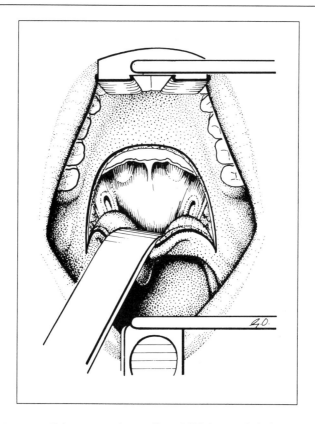

Figure 14.6   Exposure of the post-nasal space (from RSN, by permission)

5.   External facial incisions

The incisions for approach to the paranasal sinuses are shown in Figure 14.3. Facial incisions should be marked out with surgical ink to facilitate good wound apposition at the end of the procedure. If there is any risk of corneal abrasion during paranasal sinus surgery a temporary tarsorrhaphy should be performed. External frontal ethmoidectomy, ligation of the anterior ethmoidal artery and maxillectomy are discussed in subsequent chapters. The lateral rhinotomy is the workhorse of approaches to the paranasal sinuses and nasal cavity and will be discussed here in further detail.

LATERAL RHINOTOMY

Indications

A lateral rhinotomy incision provides excellent exposure to one side of the nasal cavity plus the ethmoid and maxillary sinuses. It is suitable for removal of both benign and malignant intranasal tumours and allows the surgeon to remove the entire lateral nasal wall and nasal septum if necessary. These structures may also be removed to provide deeper access.

Specimen

This will depend on the pathology being treated.

Pre-operative considerations

As with all paranasal sinus surgery, the appropriate investigations and scans should be available prior to surgery.

Risks

1. Unsightly scarring. This can be reduced by careful placement of the incision and correct repair. Similarly, vestibular stenosis should be avoided by careful surgery.
2. Epiphora. This can occur from damage to the nasolacrimal duct.
3. Haemorrhage from an uncontrolled vessel within the paranasal sinuses.
4. Cavity infection from infected crusts.
5. Facial anaesthesia from damage to the infraorbital nerve.

Preparation

Preparation of the nasal lining with vasoconstrictive agents. General oral endotracheal anaesthesia with a throat pack. The patient is supine on the table with a head ring for stability. A temporary tarsorrhaphy is performed. The entire face should be exposed. Preliminary vasoconstrictive infiltration in the line of incision is helpful.

Method

1. The upper end of the incision commences halfway between the medial canthus and the bridge of the nose. Placing a thumb over the eye often helps to identify the upper point of this incision. The incision should then run just medial to the nasomaxillary groove and run into the alar groove prior to finishing within the nasal cavity. The incision is deepened through all layers with freeing of the alar cartilage of the nose to allow retraction of the nose medially and allowing the surgeon a clear view into the nasal cavity. It can often be useful at the upper end of the incision to commence the incision through the skin and then use an artery clip to identify the angular vein. This often prevents excessive bleeding. The incision can be seen in Figure 14.3.
2. The further access and the precise procedure performed is now determined by the pathology present. The skin and periosteum overlying the nasal

bone is elevated prior to removal of part of these bones with bone nibblers or punch forceps. This bone removal can, if required, be extended to include both the lacrimal bone and lamina papyracea. This allows removal of the ethmoidal labyrinth.

3. The soft tissue of the cheek can be retracted laterally as far as the level of the infra-orbital foramen and the maxillary sinus opened and inspected. The mucosa can be removed from the maxillary sinus.

4. The nasal mucosa can be sleeved by subperiosteal dissection through a lateral rhinotomy incision and it is then possible to remove the entire lateral nasal wall as required. If the cavity is going to be packed post-operatively it is often well worthwhile to remove all bone or sharp edges within a lateral rhinotomy cavity. This can often be performed easily with the use of a diamond paste burr. Some surgeons use the drill to remove the nasal bones and parts of the frontonasal process of the maxilla in preference to the use of punch forceps.

5. The surgery performed within the nasal and paranasal sinus cavities will determine whether a post-operative pack is required.

6. The wound is closed in two layers with 4-0 chromic catgut to remove tension from the skin and 5-0 prolene or nylon to the skin.

Post-operative care

1. If a pack has been inserted then its removal will be determined by the precise nature of the operation.

2. Crusting is frequently a problem following creation of a paranasal sinus cavity. Regular cleaning is required in the first few post-operative days. A large aural speculum and the use of the operating microscope with suction can be helpful in keeping the cavity clear. It is also helpful to have a spray mechanism to keep the cavity moist and prevent dry hard crusts from forming.

3. The skin sutures should be removed after 4–5 days. The extent of post-operative regular follow-up will be determined by the state of any cavity created and the precise pathological diagnosis.

Chapter 15

Septal, turbinate and rhinoplasty surgery

SEPTAL SURGERY

Indications

Septal surgery is most often performed to correct a nasal obstruction that arises from a deformity/deviation of the nasal septum. Other indications include:

1. To improve the access to one side of the nasal cavity in order to:
   - remove nasal polyps
   - control a difficult posterior epistaxis
   - facilitate the removal of a foreign body or rhinolith.
2. To realign the septal cartilage when there is cosmetic deformity of the external cartilaginous profile.

Pre-operative considerations

A submucous resection (SMR) is removal of deviated septal cartilage or bone after first elevating mucoperiosteal/mucoperichondrial flaps. A columellar dislocation requires a septoplasty and deviations of the cartilaginous profile can also be improved by a septoplasty. When a rhinoplasty is combined with septal surgery it is considered that a septoplasty reduces septal scarring, producing a better rhinoplasty result.

There is often disagreement between surgeons as to what constitutes a septoplasty versus an SMR in current rhinological practice, particularly when only limited areas of deviated septum are removed as for our description of an SMR. Our description of septoplasty describes mobilization of the quadrilateral cartilage and reposition into the anterior columella.

Risks

1. A slight supratip depression is common following septal surgery.

2. Septal perforation is the commonest complication, producing significant symptoms.
3. Intra-nasal adhesions.
4. Complications of nasal packs.
5. Complications of nasal splints.
6. Late recurrence of nasal obstruction due to recurrence of septal deviation.
7. Septal haematoma and abscess.

Preparation

General per-oral endotracheal anaesthesia with a throat pack.

The anaesthetic tube is placed ideally in the mid line and care taken that the securing adhesive tapes do not pull unevenly on the skin of the nose. Head-up tilt is helpful. A topical vasoconstrictive agent is applied prior to transfer to the operating room and vasoconstrictive infiltration used at the time of surgery.

Septal surgery can be performed under local anaesthetic with the agents discussed in Chapter 2 (local anaesthesia) and Chapter 14 (principles of nasal surgery).

Method: submucous resection (SMR)

1. A unilateral subperichondrial incision is placed on the side of maximum septal deviation approximately 1 cm posterior to the anterior margin of the septal cartilage. Undermining the anterior edge of the incision at this stage will facilitate the suturing of the incision at the end of operation (Figure 15.1).

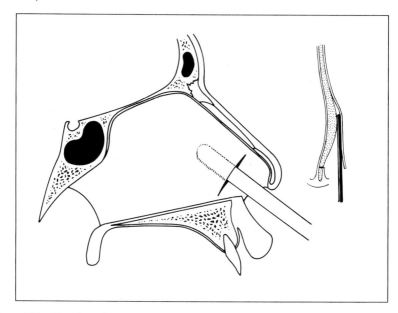

Figure 15.1 Elevation of septal mucoperiosteal flap (from RSN, by permission)

2. A mucoperichondrial flap is elevated on the side of the incision. An area of adhesion with minor bleeding will occur at the osseocartilaginous septal junction as the flap progresses into a mucoperiosteal flap. The flap is elevated, on a broad front, until the deviated part of the septum is revealed.
3. A scalpel incises a vertical score in the septal cartilage at the level of the initial incision and then a Freer's knife is used to complete the incision and enter the subperichondrial plane on the opposite side of the septal cartilage. Great care must be taken with the cartilage split incision. First, it is important to ensure that an anterior cartilage strut of at least 5–10 mm is conserved to support the septal tip. Secondly, the technique of dividing the septal cartilage should avoid dividing the mucosa on the opposite side of the septum. If an incision penetrates the full thickness of the septum it should be identified and repaired. The subperichondrial/periosteal flap is elevated on the second side.

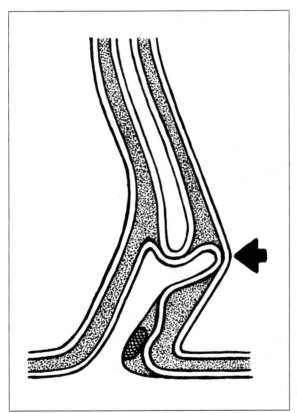

Figure 15.2 Creating a subperiosteal tunnel alongside the maxillary crest

4. If the maxillary crest is involved in the septal deviation then the mucoperiosteal flaps have to be elevated from it. This can be achieved by continuing the flap dissection from the septal direction after excising the deviated cartilage and bone. An alternative technique is to dissect on to the anterior

nasal spine with sharp pointed scissors or scalpel and then to create a tunnel alongside the maxillary crest. This tunnel is joined to the septal flaps by dividing from posterior and inferior to anterior. Figure 15.2 highlights the point that there is discontinuity of the subperiosteal layer at the apex of the maxillary crest.

5. After the flaps are elevated from the septum, the deformities can be excised. Some surgeons excise deviated septum at the same time as elevating the flaps, whereas other surgeons wait until the flaps are fully elevated and then resect the deviated septum. Only deviated septum is removed and a support strut is left at the columella and at the dorsum, which should be approximately 1 cm wide, although in experienced hands this may be reduced to 5 mm.

6. The flaps are replaced to the mid line and the initial incision may be closed with an absorbable suture. Light packing with Vaseline gauze or packing within finger cots helps oppose the septal flaps in the initial phase. Often no packs are required.

Method: septoplasty

1. A Cottle's clamp is applied to the columellar soft tissue and the columella is manipulated to present the dislocated anterior border of the quadrilateral cartilage into whichever nostril is easier. A vertical incision is placed down the anterior border of the quadrilateral cartilage. A pair of sharp pointed curved scissors is used to enter the correct subperichondrial plane. The subperichondrial flap is elevated on one side of the septum.

2. The sharp pointed curved scissors are used to delineate and enter the subperichondrial plane on the second side. It is often easier to commence the flap elevation from the superior part of the incision.

3. At this point it is useful to re-create the columellar 'groove'. The sharp pointed scissors are used to create the groove or pocket in which to place the septum at the end of the operation.

4. The flap is elevated from the second side of the septum. Dissection with sharp pointed curved scissors on to the anterior nasal spine allows the creation of subperiosteal tunnels along each side of the maxillary crest as shown in Figure 15.2. A 'hockey stick' Freer's knife used from posteroinferior to anterior is useful to create continuity between the tunnels and the main septal flaps. A scalpel can also be used to join the tunnels to the flaps.

5. It is now possible to mobilize the quadrilateral cartilage fully. Posteriorly a Freer's straight elevator is inserted into the junction between the cartilage and the bone of the perpendicular plate of the ethmoid and vomer. An angled Freer's knife elevates the cartilage from the maxillary crest and the point of a Hill's elevator is run along the junctions between the dorsal border of the quadrilateral cartilage and each upper lateral cartilage. The quadrilateral cartilage can now be potentially positioned in the mid line. The bony septum is nibbled backward until there is no overlap of cartilage on bone. Any deviated bone is also removed. Gross deviations of the maxillary crest are removed. The removal of an inferior sliver of septal cartilage may facilitate the cartilage reposition. This is shown in Figure

15.3. Scoring and cross hatch techniques are often used to help position the septum in the mid line, although many surgeons believe that full cartilaginous mobilization is the most important factor.

6. The mucoperichondrial flaps are replaced. A mattress transfixion suture can be useful to secure flaps. The initial incision is closed with an absorbable suture and the nostrils may be lightly packed with Vaseline gauze or packing within finger cots to help oppose the flaps.

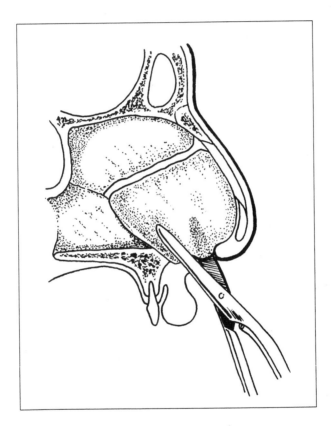

Figure 15.3   Removal of inferior sliver of cartilage from the quadrilateral plate (from RSN, by permission)

Post-operative care

Packing is generally removed after 24 hours and the patient usually leaves hospital within the following 48 hours. Steam inhalations can be helpful while some surgeons decrust the nostril margin and apply a mild antiseptic cream within the nares.

Specific problems at septal surgery

1.   The full thickness perforation of the septum

This unfortunate situation means that a septal perforation is the likely outcome. If it is technically possible the tears should be repaired with absorbable sutures. When this is not possible a piece of resected cartilage should be 'straightened' in a cartilage press and inserted between the flaps to support the mucosa and allow closure. If possible a mattress suture placed through the flaps and the cartilage will hold the cartilage graft in place.

2.   Excessive bleeding during the raising of the flaps

A superficial plane that has been entered is the likely explanation. Scraping the cartilage will often demonstrate a thin membrane under which the correct subperichondrial plane lies.

3.   A tear in the flap on the same side as surgery of the inferior turbinate

The danger exists here of an adhesion between the septum and the inferior turbinate. A silastic splint for 7 to 10 days will prevent the formation of an adhesion. Some surgeons do not insert splints and arrange a weekly review to divide any filmy adhesion.

4.   Sutures keep tearing out during closure of the initial incision

Some surgeons do not close the incision for an SMR. If the incision does not lie easily together a small area of uncomfortable granulation can develop. When the sutures tear out a small silastic splint will help to allow the unsutured incision to sit evenly.

5.   Septal haematoma

Following surgery, the factor that often first brings a septal haematoma to notice is increasing pain over the dorsum and at the columella of the nose. A swelling of the septum may be found, although it is important to realize that mild septal oedema and local discomfort follows septal surgery. Needle aspiration will confirm the diagnosis. Parenteral antibiotics are required to prevent septal abscess and a definitive drainage procedure is preferable to repeated aspiration. The opening of the incision and insertion of a small tube drain is appropriate.

6.   Nasal splint insertion

It is important that a nasal splint should lie alongside the septum! (Figure 15.4). Care should be taken that the superior border of the splint does not lie lateral to the inferior or middle turbinate as this can cause great discomfort. The splint in correct position should move easily in an antero-posterior direction. The splint should be secured to its neighbour on the other side or taped to the cheek to prevent inhalation.

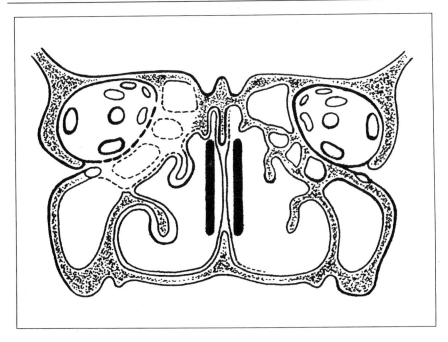

Figure 15.4 Splints alongside the nasal septum

SUBMUCOUS DIATHERMY TO THE INFERIOR TURBINATE

Indications

Nasal obstruction due to turbinate enlargement. Excessive rhinorrhoea in vasomotor rhinitis. Recent research has called into question the value of this operation, as a significant number of patients have a recurrence of symptoms within a year.

Risks

1. Intra-nasal adhesions.
2. Epistaxis.
3. Failure of symptoms to improve.
4. Injury to orbital contents has been reported.

Preparation

General oral endotracheal anaesthesia with a throat pack. Head-up tilt is helpful. A topical nasal vasoconstrictive agent is applied.

Method

1. A pointed electrode which is insulated except for 5 mm at the tip is connected to a standard unipolar coagulation diathermy source with the earth electrode applied to the upper thigh.
2. A nasal speculum is used to reveal the anterior end of the inferior turbinate. The electrode is placed against the anterior surface of the inferior turbinate and a brief closure of the electric circuit cauterizes the point of entry.
3. The electrode is inserted through the length of the inferior turbinate parallel to the floor of the nose. Care is taken to prevent buttonholing the turbinate mucosa. The diathermy circuit is completed and the electrode slowly withdrawn through the turbinate. Up to three passes of the electrode through the turbinate should be applied. This is shown in Figure 15.5.
4. Only if there is considerable bleeding is a nasal pack required.

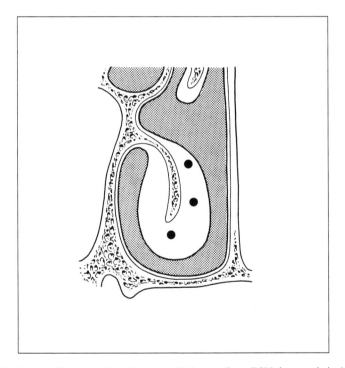

Figure 15.5   Points of insertion for submucous diathermy (from RSN, by permission)

Post-operative care

1. If the mucosa has been grossly buttonholed or the surgeon considers that there is a risk of an intranasal adhesion for another reason it is advisable to review the patient after 7 days to identify and divide any adhesion.

2. The patient usually leaves hospital the day after surgery. There is initial mucosal swelling and the patient will often not start to feel improvement until about a month after the operation.

TURBINECTOMY

Indications for inferior turbinectomy

1. Nasal obstruction due to a hypertrophic inferior turbinate.
2. Removal of the anterior end of the inferior turbinate can facilitate the creation of an intra-nasal antrostomy.
3. A tumour involving the inferior turbinate.

Indications for middle turbinectomy

1. To assist drainage from the middle meatus and the frontonasal duct.
2. A tumour involving the middle turbinate.

Pre-operative considerations

All turbinate tissue is very vascular and in particular removal of the entire inferior turbinate can be followed by severe haemorrhage. The use of unipolar diathermy applied through the submucous diathermy needle can be helpful in reducing bleeding. If there is excessive bleeding then an adequate nasal pack should be inserted at the time of surgery.

Any history of bleeding disorders should be identified pre-operatively and investigated haematologically.

Risks

1. Atrophic rhinitis may occasionally follow a radical turbinectomy with the nose becoming widely patent, dry, crusting and uncomfortable. This can occur especially if a turbinectomy is combined with an inferior meatal antrostomy.
2. Post-operative haemorrhage.
3. Complete removal and loss of the landmark of the middle turbinate will make any subsequent ethmoid sinus surgery more hazardous.

Preparation

General per-oral endotracheal anaesthesia with a throat pack. Head-up tilt is helpful. A topical nasal vasoconstrictive agent is applied.

Method: anterior end inferior turbinate

A cut is made with turbinate scissors for 13 mm back from the anterior end of the turbinate. A cutting snare is used to remove the piece with the cut oblique so that the anterior end of the inferior turbinate slopes backwards. Exposed turbinate bone may have to be trimmed (Figure 15.6).

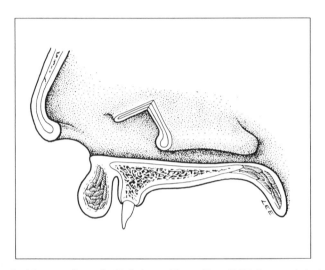

Figure 15.6   Excision anterior end of inferior turbinate (from RSN, by permission)

Method: posterior end inferior turbinate

A nasal cutting snare is used with the wire slightly angled. The snare is inserted past the posterior end of the turbinate and withdrawn until it loops around the tissue to be removed (Figure 15.7). Closure of the snare separates the posterior end of the turbinate which can then be picked from the nose with a pair of Tilly Henckel forceps. When the snare cannot be used the posterior end can be grasped with a Luc's forceps and removed by pushing backwards into the nasopharynx.

Method: the entire inferior turbinate

A polypoid fringe of inferior turbinate can be removed with a pair of turbinate scissors (Figure 15.8). The removal of the entire turbinate is performed by first dislocating the inferior turbinate medially with an instrument such as a Hill's elevator and then using a pair of turbinectomy scissors to divide the turbinate from its lateral attachment.

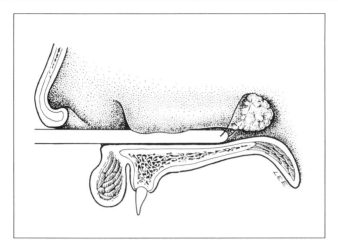

Figure 15.7   Excision posterior end of inferior turbinate (from RSN, by permission)

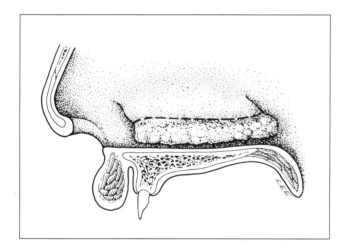

Figure 15.8   Polypoid fringe excision from the inferior turbinate (from RSN, by permission)

Method: the middle turbinate

A cut is made with turbinate scissors from the antero-superior margin of the middle turbinate in a posterior direction. A cutting snare can then be insinuated over the anterior end of the turbinate and the appropriate amount of tissue removed.

Reduction of a concha bullosa is described under Functional endoscopic sinus surgery (Chapter 17).

Post-operative care

The nasal pack is usually removed after 24 hours and the patient discharged the following day.

RHINOPLASTY

Introduction

A poor rhinoplasty result is obvious and often difficult to correct. Observation of an expert surgeon plus operation under supervision is mandatory prior to a surgeon attempting a 'solo' rhinoplasty.

Indications

Variation from a well-proportioned straight nose may be considered an indication for rhinoplasty in a particular individual. A reduction rhinoplasty is usually indicated in a patient with a larger than normal nose with a prominent nasal hump. The basic reduction rhinoplasty technique will be described in the following sections. When the deviation of the nasal pyramid plays a large part in nasal obstruction in association with a septal deviation then a septo-rhinoplasty may be required. The medial and lateral osteotomies as described below for the basic reduction rhinoplasty in addition to the septoplasty procedure constitute the basic techniques for the septorhinoplasty.

Pre-operative considerations

1. Prior to a rhinoplasty it is important that both the surgeon and the patient are aware of the limitations of the surgery to be performed. A very good question to ask a patient is 'Tell me exactly what features of your nose you would like altered?' In general a patient will tell you exactly what he or she wants and it is then possible to discuss the likely outcome of surgery. Occasionally, however, patients may give very vague explanations of the alterations they wish to their nose or suggest that nasal surgery will result in a tremendous alteration to their sex appeal or ability to make money. It is wise, for the latter patient, to obtain a second opinion either from another nasal surgeon or a psychiatrist!
2. The appearance of a nose can be classified from 1 to 5, with number 1 being perfect and number 5 being very unattractive. It is reasonable to expect an improvement by one place, i.e. a number 3 to a number 2, but unreasonable to expect an improvement from a number 5 to a number 1.
3. The surgeon should identify the anatomical factors which constitute the deformity and be able to define mentally the steps which will be required to correct the deformity.
4. Good pre-operative photographs are mandatory for medico-legal reasons to allow the patient and the surgeon to discuss the proposed changes and to

be placed on the X-ray box in the operating room for reference during the actual surgery.

Risks

1. Anaesthesia over bridge of the nose.
2. Bruising under the eyes which rarely can lead to permanent under-eye discoloration.
3. Local abscess in the nose.
4. Failure to correct the deformity fully.

Preparation

1. A nasal topical vasoconstrictive agent is applied.
2. General anaesthesia is delivered through an oral cuffed endotracheal tube with a protective throat pack inserted. The tube is placed in the mid line and care taken that the securing adhesive tapes do not pull unevenly on the skin of the nose.
3. The eyes are protected with Steri-Strip tapes placed across the lateral corners of the eyelids. Care is taken with the positioning of the head towels and the eye tapes so that there is no uneven pull on the nasal skin.
4. Head-up tilt is important to reduce nasal venous congestion.
5. A local anaesthetic vasoconstrictive agent is injected (see Chapter 3, Local Anaesthesia, and Chapter 14, Principles of Nasal Surgery). The sites of injection include:
   - Between the upper lateral and lower lateral cartilages.
   - Along the nasal dorsum.
   - Into the region of the infraorbital nerve.
   - Along the site of the lateral osteotomy.
   - Along the columella.
   - Along the lower margin of the lower lateral cartilage.
   - Under the mucoperichondrium of the septum if an associated septo-plasty is to be performed.
6. Rhinoplasty can be performed under local anaesthetic with sedation. The local anaesthetic agents in Chapter 3 are appropriate.
7. The nasal hairs are trimmed to permit the optimal visibility of the operation site. This can be performed while awaiting the vasoconstrictive agents to take effect.

Method

1. An alar retractor is used to elevate the nasal rim and external pressure from the index finger over the upper lateral cartilage defines the line between the upper and lower lateral cartilages in which the intercartilaginous incision is placed. The incision is created with a number 15 scalpel and continued medially to become continuous with the transfixion incision which separates the columella flush from the caudal border of the

nasal septum. The line of the intercartilaginous incision is shown in Figure 15.9.

2. The skin overlying the upper nasal cartilages and the nasal bones is elevated either with a pair of curved blunt-ended scissors or with a number 15 scalpel. The skin elevation should extend to just beyond the glabella, but not on to the forehead.

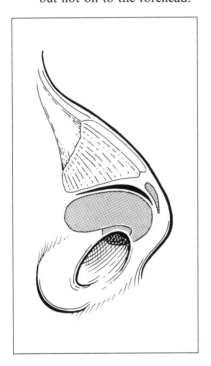

Figure 15.9   Site of intercartilaginous incision (from RSN, by permission)

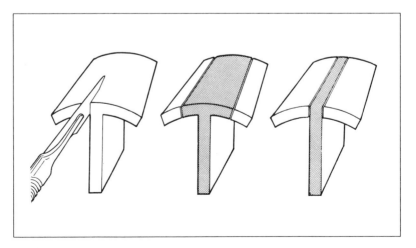

Figure 15.10   Division of upper lateral cartilage (from RSN, by permission)

3. A periosteal elevator is used to elevate the periosteum from the nasal bones. Care is taken that the upper lateral cartilage is not disarticulated from the nasal bones.
4. The upper lateral cartilages are divided at their medial attachment to the nasal septum (Figure 15.10). An Aufrecht's retractor protects the skin of the nasal dorsum and provides excellent exposure to allow an accurate division to be performed flush with the nasal septum either with a number 11 blade scalpel or with heavy straight scissors (Mayo).

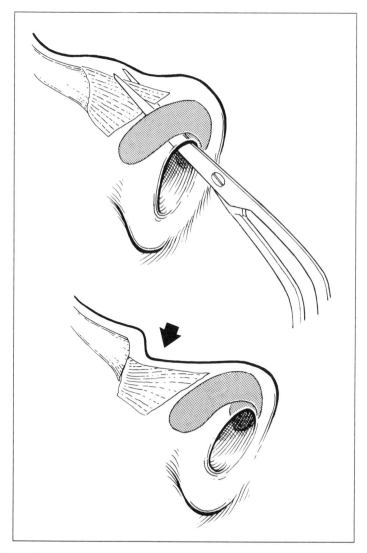

Figure 15.11   Step deformity after lowering of cartilaginous nasal hump (from RSN, by permission)

5.   The nasal septum and the upper lateral cartilages are lowered, one at a time, with a pair of Foman scissors up to the bony nasal hump. This results in an obvious step deformity which can be seen if the profile of the nose is viewed from the lateral aspect (Figure 15.11).

6.   The bony nasal hump is lowered either with a T-shaped chisel (Figure 15.12) or a wide straight chisel. The bar of the T chisel allows the surgeon to identify the plane of his or her cut and to prevent an excess removal of bone from one side. A wide chisel is required to ensure that the entire width of the hump is removed and to prevent dangerous tunnelling with a narrow osteotome. The bony hump is grasped with a pair of heavy artery forceps and should be advanced further into the nose prior to removal in order to divide any connection between the mucous membrane, periosteum and bone. A rasp is inserted to smooth and even the nasal bones and bony nasal septum.

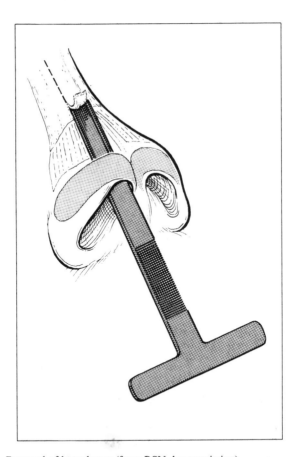

Figure 15.12   Removal of bony hump (from RSN, by permission)

7.   A wide 10–13 mm osteotome is used to create the two medial osteotomies. A narrow osteotome may slip under the nasal bones and penetrate through the cribriform plate. On each occasion the osteotome is inserted

alongside the nasal septum until it engages the inferior margin of the nasal bones. A very slight lateral curve as the osteotome ascends may produce a more natural root to the nose because on in-fracture the nasal bones will come to lie under the remaining bony spine (Figure 15.13).

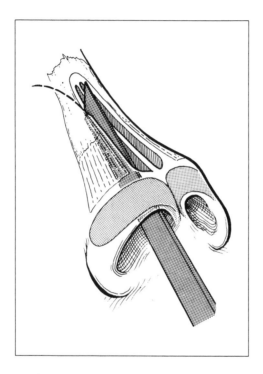

Figure 15.13 Medial osteotomies (from RSN, by permission)

8. Lateral osteotomies may be performed either externally or internally. There are expert proponents of each technique. External lateral osteotomies are performed through external stab incisions (usually two a side) with a 2 mm osteotome (Figure 15.14). Internal lateral osteotomies are performed through the pyriform aperture and are curved towards the medial osteotomies to avoid the need for a superior osteotomy. It is important that the lateral osteotomies are placed close to the face to prevent a step deformity as shown in Figure 15.15. The nasal bones are infractured and the profile of the nose is reassessed to ensure the hump deformity of cartilage and bone has been corrected equally.

9. The modification of the nasal tip requires meticulous technique, particularly in patients with thin skin as mistakes can be very obvious. Care should be taken not to damage the cosmetically important lower margin of the lower lateral cartilage. The objective of the technique described here is to excise the upper border of the lower lateral cartilage as depicted in Figure 15.16. The lower border of the lower lateral cartilage is not parallel to the lower margin of the nasal rim but ascends as it sweeps laterally.

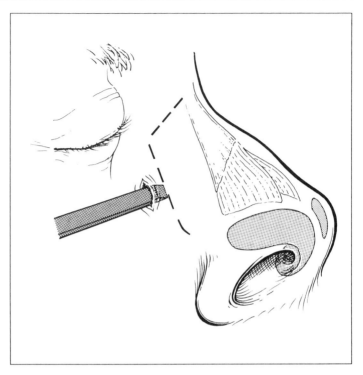

Figure 15.14   External lateral osteotomies (from RSN, by permission)

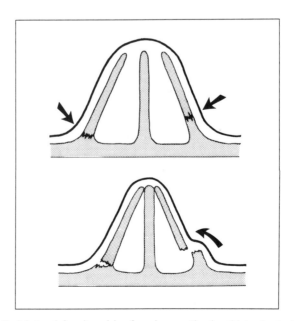

Figure 15.15   Facial step deformity arising from incorrectly placed lateral osteotomy (from RSN, by permission)

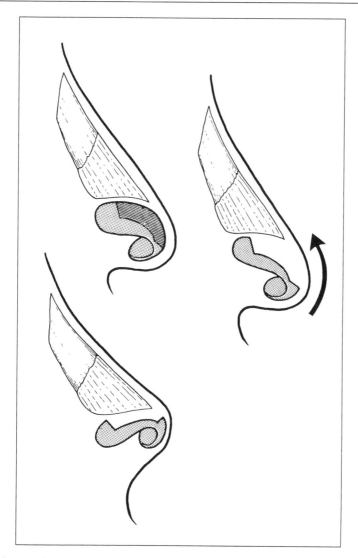

Figure 15.16 Refinement of the nasal tip (from RSN, by permission)

This margin can often be identified at the junction between the hair bearing and non-hair bearing vestibular skin and should be palpated prior to the cartilage splitting incision.

10. The incision is placed to leave an intact lower rim of cartilage approximately 2–3 mm wide. Sharp pointed scissors are inserted through the cartilage splitting incision and elevate the skin overlying the upper part of the lower lateral cartilage. The lower margin of the upper part of the lower lateral cartilage is grasped in a pair of fine toothed forceps and a Freer's elevator is insinuated through the cartilage splitting incision and

out through the intercartilaginous incision. This exposes and allows the appropriate segment of cartilage to be excised. Excessive damage to the vestibular skin can lead to scarring and pinched in appearance at the nasal vestibule.

11. Removal of the upper segment of the lower lateral cartilage mildly rotates upwards the nasal tip and slightly shortens the nose as well as removing bulkiness from the nasal tip. When judging the line of the cartilage splitting incision it is possible to increase or decrease the tip projection by leaving or removing the cartilage medial to the dome.

12. All the incisions are closed with a fine (4/0) absorbable suture on an atraumatic needle and the nose is firmly packed internally prior to application of the external dressing and plaster.

13. Broad Steri-Strips are placed across the dorsum of the nose and around the tip of the nose as shown in Figure 15.17. There should be no gap between the Steri-Strips as this can result in skin herniation and a resultant necrotic strip of skin. A plaster cast is applied on top of the Steri-Strips. During the application of the external splint it is important to ensure that any blood which has collected under the skin is expressed through the incisions.

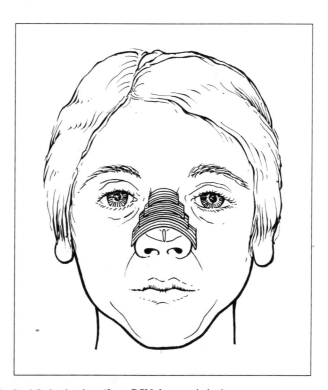

Figure 15.17   Steri-Strips in place (from RSN, by permission)

Post-operative care

1. The patient should be sat up post-operatively and ice packs may be required if there is an excess of bruising along the line of the lateral osteotomy.
2. Nasal packing is removed between 24 and 48 hours and the patient discharged the following day.
3. The external nasal splint is removed after 7–14 days, at which time the first in a series of post-operative photographs should be taken.

EXTERNAL APPROACH RHINOPLASTY

Indications

An external approach to the nose allows the surgeon excellent exposure and visibility of the external skeleton and soft tissue of the nose. This permits accurate correction of lower lateral cartilage deformities such as alar valve augmentation and can be very helpful when performing a septorhinoplasty on a severely traumatized nose. Small cysts (i.e. sebaceous cyst) and tumours which affect the nasal tip and dorsum of the nose can also be removed through an external approach. It is important, however, to realize that the external approach only improves access prior to the performance of standard rhinoplastic techniques.

Risks

1. Those of any rhinoplasty.
2. Very minimal problems have been encountered in the cosmesis of the columellar incision particularly in the hands of a precise and experienced surgeon.

Preparation

In addition to the usual preparation for a rhinoplasty the external incision should be carefully marked out with surgical ink (including 'cross marks' to permit matching up the incision at closure) prior to infiltration of the nasal tip with vasoconstrictive solution. A dry field is crucial for the incision of the external approach.

Method

1. Figure 15.18 demonstrates the incision for an external approach. The transverse part of the incision is placed at the mid point of the columella and has the V notch placed in it to disguise and minimize the effect of the final scar. A number 11 scalpel creates the transverse incision and then runs

laterally on each side along the inferior margins of the lower lateral cartilage (lateral crus).

2. A fine skin hook picks up the upper flap of the columella and with a pair of fine pointed sharp scissors the skin is elevated from the medial and lateral crus of the lower lateral cartilages. A sterile cotton bud can be helpful in keeping the surgical field dry during the approach. As the skin is elevated the suspensory ligament of the nose is encountered and this should be divided prior to elevating the skin of the external nose with a pair of curved blunt pointed scissors. This completes the approach.
3. Standard rhinoplasty techniques are used.
4. Closure of the incisions should be performed meticulously with extra fine (6/0 catgut) within the nostril and fine monofilament externally (6/0 proline).

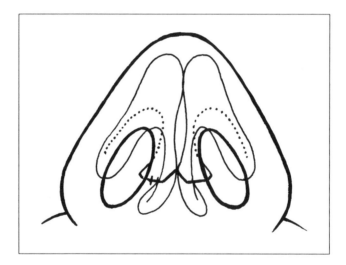

Figure 15.18   The stepped columellar incision (solid line) continuing into the dotted rim incision which follows the line of the lower edge of the lower lateral cartilage

Post-operative care

This should be as for any rhinoplasty. The non-absorbable sutures are removed after 4 to 5 days.

Chapter 16

Surgery of the maxilla

INTRA-NASAL ANTROSTOMY

Indications

An intra-nasal antrostomy may be appropriate for cases of simple sub-acute or chronic empyema of the maxillary sinus in which the diagnosis has been confirmed, but the condition has not been cured by one or two proof punctures with lavage. This route may be used, on occasion, to perform a biopsy on a suspected neoplastic lesion.

Specimen

Some material may be sent for bacteriological or histological examination.

Pre-operative considerations

In some instances functional endoscopic surgery may be considered to correct an abnormality within the osteomeatal complex which predisposes to an empyema of the maxillary sinus.

Risks

1. Epistaxis from the sphenopalatine artery.
2. Nasolacrimal duct damage.
3. Early closure of the antrostomy.
4. Failure to relieve the patient's symptoms.
5. Damage to the infra-orbital nerve.

Preparation

General peroral endotracheal anaesthesia with a throat pack. Head-up tilt is helpful. A topical vasoconstriction agent is applied to the nasal lining on the ward or after the induction of anaesthesia and before the operation. The operation can be performed under local anaesthetic with sedation.

Method

1. The inferior turbinate is dislocated medially either with a Hill's elevator or by inserting and opening a long bladed Killian's nasal speculum lateral to the inferior turbinate.
2. The initial opening is created with the point of the Hill's elevator or a similar perforating instrument (Figure 16.1). The opening is enlarged posteriorly with Luc's punch forceps and anteriorly with Ostrum's back-biting forceps (Figure 16.2). The edges should be accurately punched out.

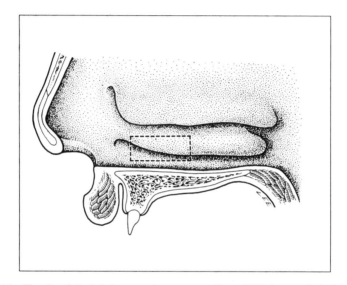

Figure 16.1   The site of the inferior meatal antrostomy (from RSN, by permission)

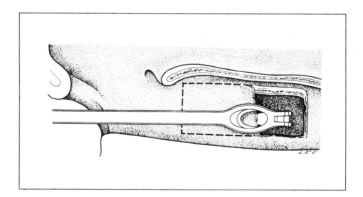

Figure 16.2   Enlarging the intranasal antrostomy anteriorly (from RSN, by permission)

3. The antrostomy should extend to the nasal floor and as far forward as possible to permit easy cannulation of the maxillary sinus. The descending branch of the sphenopalatine artery with consequent severe haemorrhage

will be encountered if the antrostomy is created too far back in the nose. A very high and anterior antrostomy may damage the nasolacrimal duct leading to subsequent stenosis and epiphora.
4. The nose is lightly packed if there is bleeding at the end of the operation.

Post-operative care

Any packing is removed the following day and steam inhalations or warm saline irrigations are used to facilitate the clearing of the maxillary sinus.

CALDWELL–LUC AND RELATED OPERATIONS

Caldwell–Luc procedure: indications

A Caldwell–Luc opening of the anterior surface of the maxilla is a good approach to inspect the contents of the maxillary paranasal sinus. The opening facilitates:

1. The removal of the mucosal lining of the maxillary antrum in 'chronic hyperplastic sinusitis'.
2. The removal of intra-sinus foreign bodies (tooth roots).
3. The inspection and biopsy of a 'tumour'.
4. The closure of an oroantral fistula.
5. The removal of intra-sinus dental cysts.
6. The removal of an antrochoanal polyp, particularly if the cyst has recurred following intra-nasal removal.

The route through the maxillary sinus from a Caldwell–Luc procedure affords access through the posterior wall of the maxillary sinus to the pterygopalatine fossa for procedures on the internal maxillary artery, maxillary division of the trigeminal nerve and the Vidian nerve. The floor of the orbit can be inspected through the maxillary antrum and procedures such as decompression of the orbital contents or repair of an infra-orbital blow-out fracture can be performed. The ethmoidal air cells can be approached and opened through the maxillary sinus (Jansen–Horgan operation). Continuation through this route allows exploration of the sphenoid sinus and pituitary fossa.

Specimen

This will depend on the precise indication for the procedure.

Pre-operative considerations

A Caldwell–Luc procedure should not be performed until after the eruption of the secondary dentition to avoid unnecessary damage. Prior to a Caldwell–Luc procedure a patient should be warned of the possibility of post-operative numbness of the cheek from stretch to the infra-orbital nerve. Patients who wear upper dentures should be aware that they may not be able to wear the dentures in the immediate post-operative period and on occasion may require the denture to be remade.

Risks

1. Cheek anaesthesia from damage to the infra-orbital nerve.
2. Poor fit of dentures.
3. Damage to dental roots with subsequent death of teeth.
4. Oroantral fistula.
5. Epistaxis from the sphenopalatine artery.
6. Nasolacrimal duct damage.
7. Early closure of the antrostomy.
8. Failure to relieve the patient's symptoms.

Preparation

General peroral endotracheal anaesthesia with a throat pack. Head-up tilt is helpful. A topical vasoconstrictive agent can be applied to the nasal lining on the ward or after the induction of anaesthesia and before the operation. The sublabial tissues are infiltrated with a vasoconstrictive solution. Care must be taken with the quantity of anaesthetic and vasoconstrictive agents used. The operation can be performed under local anaesthetic with sedation.

Method

1. The upper lip is retracted and the incision is placed immediately superior to the line of gingivolabial reflection. The incision commences at the anterior margin of the first molar tooth and runs medially to the canine ridge. The soft tissues are incised down to bone and then a heavy periosteal elevator is used to elevate the soft tissues from the anterior face of the maxilla. Figure 16.3 shows the start of a Caldwell–Luc procedure. Care should be taken that the elevation of the soft tissue stops short of the infra-orbital foramen and nerve! Haemostasis is secured with coagulation diathermy prior to entering the antrum.
2. A small gouge may be used to remove a morsel of anterior wall bone while preserving the integrity of the mucosal lining. Hajek's sphenoidal punch forceps can be used to enlarge the opening into the sinus. The opening into the sinus should be approximately 1.5 cm in diameter. A tearing action with large punch forceps should be avoided as a fracture line into the infra-orbital foramen and consequent damage to the infra-orbital nerve can occur from this technique.
3. Bony removal too far medially will encounter a heavy buttress of bone. Bony removal too far laterally will often produce an increase in the bleeding. Bony removal to the level of the antral floor risks damage to the roots of the teeth.

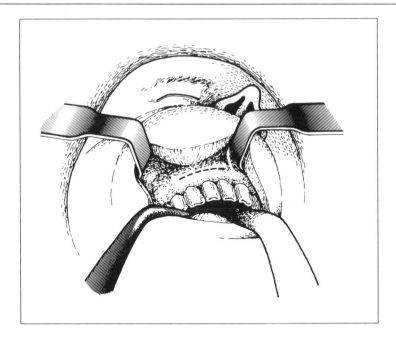

Figure 16.3 The sublabial incision (from RSN, by permission)

4. An alternative method of creating the opening into the maxillary antrum is with a cutting burr and an air drill. A fine cutting burr can be used to outline the window, which can then be elevated free with a periosteal elevator. A large burr can smooth the margins of the window.
5. The antral mucosa is incised and the contents of the sinus inspected. The mucosal lining is usually removed and this is performed with the use of straight and curved periosteal elevators. Removal of the mucosal lining intact can reduce the problem of bleeding. Should the bleeding be excessive at this part of the operation a Negus aspirating dissector, dissection with a tonsil swab, suction with a large pharyngeal sucker and coagulation diathermy can all be of use. Once the mucosal lining is stripped from the maxillary antrum the bleeding will reduce considerably. Another technique is to pack gauze tape into the antrum between the bone and the mucoperiosteal lining. As the tape is packed in it strips the lining off the bone.
6. When the indicated procedure is to treat an infective or 'chronic sinusitis' problem then an intra-nasal antrostomy is created at the end of the procedure.
7. To create the antrostomy the lateral bulge of the inferior meatus is identified and a sliver of bone removed with a gouge. The Hajek's punch forceps are useful to enlarge the bony opening into the inferior meatus. On occasion a flap of mucosa can be turned into the maxillary sinus. The edge of the antrostomy should not be rasped.
8. The antrostomy should extend to the nasal floor and as far forward as possible to permit easy cannulation of the maxillary sinus. The descending

branch of the sphenopalatine artery with consequent severe haemorrhage will be encountered if the antrostomy is created too far back in the nose. A very high anterior antrostomy may damage the nasolacrimal duct leading to subsequent stenosis and epiphora.

9.   If bleeding is a problem then the cavity can be packed with BIPP (bismuth iodoform paraffin paste) impregnated ribbon gauze with the tail of the packing led out through the antrostomy and taped to the cheek. Alternatively a balloon catheter can be inflated within the cavity and the end of the catheter taped to the cheek.

10.   The buccal wound is closed with absorbable catgut. Sufficient sutures to ensure that the wound sits evenly is all that is required.

Post-operative care

The nasal packing or catheter balloon are usually removed after 24 to 48 hours. Dentures can be fitted when the patient feels comfortable with them. The patient should start on a soft diet and work progressively to a normal diet. Steam inhalations or warm saline irrigations are useful to facilitate the clearing of the maxillary sinus.

MAXILLARY ARTERY LIGATION

Indications

Most significant nasal bleeding can be controlled by appropriate packing or local measures. In some instances, however, if the epistaxis persists for more than 3 to 4 days and the patient has required a significant blood transfusion as a result of blood loss then it is appropriate to consider maxillary artery ligation, usually combined with ethmoidal artery ligation in an attempt to control the bleeding.

It is generally believed that bleeding from above the level of the middle turbinate is considered to be anterior ethmoidal in origin while bleeding from below that to arise from the maxillary artery territory. When faced with a patient who is having severe uncontrollable epistaxis it would seem wise to ligate both anterior ethmoidal and maxillary artery on the basis that the patient may have some anatomical variant which predisposes to bleeding from one or other of the territories. Ligation of the anterior ethmoidal vessels is considered in the next chapter. In many instances bleeding from the ethmoidal area usually follows trauma. Manipulation of any nasal fracture may result in cessation of the bleeding by allowing a vessel held open by a fracture to move and go into spasm.

Vascular tumours of the nasopharynx and nose may be supplied by the maxillary artery. An example of this would be the nasopharyngeal angio-fibroma. Preliminary ligation of the maxillary artery and feeding vessels prior to extirpation of these vascular tumours is often a sensible preliminary procedure.

Some surgeons believe that there is a place for maxillary artery ligation in recurrent non-specific epistaxis and hereditary haemorrhagic telangiectasia. The evidence for this is limited.

Pre-operative considerations

Precautions as for a Caldwell–Luc procedure should be taken and the patient warned of problems of facial anaesthesia and difficulty with fitting dentures after the procedure. A patient should always be fully resuscitated before proceeding to theatre for maxillary artery ligation in cases of acute massive epistaxis and cross-matched blood should be available.

In those cases where it is the vascular supply of a tumour that is to be ligated it is appropriate to have the preliminary angiograms placed on a viewing box in theatre to facilitate the identification of the vessels for ligation. The feasibility of embolization should have been discussed with the radiologist and found to be inappropriate or unavailable.

Risks

1. Cheek anaesthesia from damage to the infra-orbital nerve.
2. Poor fit of dentures.
3. Damage to dental roots with subsequent death of teeth.
4. Oroantral fistula.
5. Epistaxis from the sphenopalatine artery.
6. Nasolacrimal duct damage.
7. Failure to control severe epistaxis from the side of the nose.

Preparation

General anaesthesia through a peroral endotracheal tube with a throat pack in place. The patient is supine on the table, head up and with a head ring under the head. The sublabial tissues are infiltrated with a vasoconstrictive solution.

Method

1. The initial surgical steps are as for a Caldwell–Luc procedure, although the anterior opening into the maxillary sinus should be made as large as is technically possible. The opening is limited superiorly by the infraorbital nerve and one must take care in removing bone inferiorly that one does not damage the apices of the teeth.
2. Once good access is available through the maxillary antrum the mucosa is removed from the posterior wall of the antrum. Small chisel cuts are used to outline an elliptical window on the thin posterior wall of the antrum. Only the bone is perforated, with care being taken to avoid penetrating the periosteal layer behind the bone.

3. A self-retaining mastoid retractor can often effectively retract the soft tissues and allow a clear view through the maxillary antrum through a microscope with a 300 mm objective lens. The window of bone is now lifted from the periosteum with a small curved elevator and removed. There is often a prominent transverse vein running across the periosteum and this can be coagulated with bipolar or unipolar diathermy.

4. The maxillary artery always lies superficial or anterior to the maxillary nerve.

5. Scissors, preferably curved on the flat with rounded ends, are inserted through the periosteum and opened widely in both the vertical and horizontal planes to provide a cruciate opening into the pterygopalatine fossa. The maxillary artery is often detectable by its pulsation and can be defined by further artery clip or scissor dissection. Figure 16.4 shows these points.

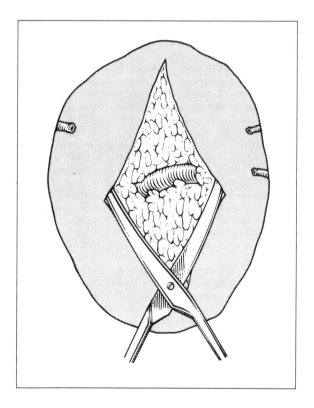

Figure 16.4   Opening the pterygopalatine fossa (from RSN, by permission)

6. A curved hook, such as a Golding-Wood hook, or failing that a St Bart's wax hook, can be used to place the vessel under slight tension to allow the separation of the artery from its surrounding fat by artery clip or scissor dissection. This exposes the full arterial pattern within the pterygopalatine fossa which is shown in Figure 16.5.

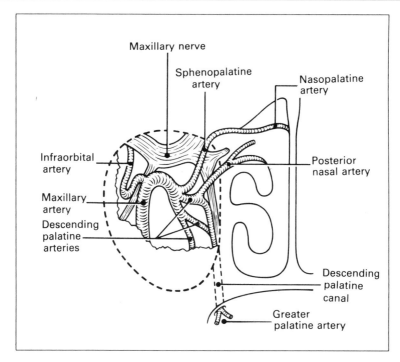

Figure 16.5 Anatomy of the maxillary artery and its branches (from RSN, by permission)

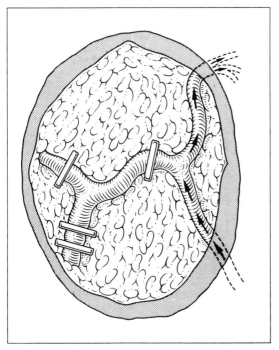

Figure 16.6 Clips on the major branches of the maxillary artery in the pterygopalatine fossa. Note the reverse of arterial flow in the unclipped vessels (from RSN, by permission)

7. With the artery held under slight tension, tantalon clips are applied to occlude both the proximal trunk and the infra-orbital branch. Two clips are placed under the proximal end of the maxillary artery for safety. It is important to attempt to clip all of the branches of the maxillary artery within the pterygopalatine fossa and one should look for them, as demonstrated in Figure 16.6.
8. Once all the clips are in place it is then wise to divide the artery between the clips.
9. If one is dealing with a severe epistaxis and the anterior ethmoidal vessel has been ligated it is worthwhile unpacking the nose at this stage. If there is still persistent oozing from the side of the nose then it is worth searching for an undivided vessel, such as an anomalous pharyngeal artery or an unidentified terminal branch of the maxillary artery. The medial part of the pterygopalatine fossa, therefore, should be explored.
10. At the completion of ligation of both the maxillary artery and anterior ethmoidal artery some surgeons may leave the side of the nose that has been bleeding unpacked. Most cautious surgeons, however, would pack the nose at the end of the procedure.
11. The buccal wound is closed with absorbable catgut. Sufficient sutures to ensure that the wound sits evenly is all that is required.

Post-operative care

The nasal packing can be removed after 24 to 48 hours. Dentures can be fitted when the patient feels comfortable with them. The patient should start on a soft diet and work progressively to a normal diet.

MAXILLECTOMY

Indications

A maxillectomy is most commonly performed as an oncological procedure in the management of maxillary tumours, of which squamous cell carcinoma is the most common.

To be an effective procedure resection must encompass the lesion. A tumour that has extended posteriorly and has eroded the pterygoid plates is generally considered irresectable. If the orbit is involved then the eye has to be removed at the initial operation. Consent for removal of the eye should always be considered when consenting a patient for maxillectomy. In some instances it is only possible to determine whether the eye can be saved at the time of the operation. If there is invasion of the tumour into the skin then the skin will have to be removed and replaced by a flap. Both the CT scan and the MRI scan have an important role in the assessment of maxillary tumours.

In rare instances severe fungal infections of the maxilla may be an indication for a maxillectomy when anti-fungal preparations have failed to control the disease.

Specimen

The maxilla, with or without the eye.

Pre-operative considerations

It is important to involve a prosthodontist prior to the operation in order that an impression can be made from either the patient's dentures or teeth so that an obturator can be designed to fill the defect left by the surgery. As mentioned above, consent for removal of the eye must be considered prior to the surgery. A cross-match of blood for 2 units is appropriate.

Risks

1. The patient has a numb cheek following this operation.
2. Post-operative haemorrhage from a partially damaged maxillary artery is always possible.
3. In some instances airway compromise can occur following a maxillectomy, particularly with a very loose fitting prosthesis. If there is any doubt as to the patient's airway post-operatively then a tracheostomy should be performed.
4. Failure to control the disease.

Preparation

General anaesthesia through a peroral endotracheal tube with a throat pack. The patient is supine, head supported on a head ring and the face well exposed after the towelling procedure. A temporary tarsorrhaphy should be performed on both eyes to protect them from inadvertent damage during surgery.

Method

1. Figure 14.3B shows the external incision and Figure 16.7 demonstrates the internal incision lines. When the orbit is to be retained then a horizontal incision passes approximately 2 mm below the lash margins along the lower eyelid. If the orbital contents are to be removed then a circumferential incision is made through the conjunctiva, which allows preservation of both eyelids and thus facilitates the fitting of an ocular prosthesis.
2. The intra-oral incision which follows the alveolar buccal sulcus allows the skin of the face to be peeled laterally from the underlying maxillary bone. The mid-line incision usually passes anteriorly in the region of the first upper incisor. If this tooth is present then it has to be removed to allow the incision to be created.
3. The facial skin and buccinator muscle are raised from the anterior wall of the maxilla back to the zygomatic arch and the lateral margin of the malar bone.

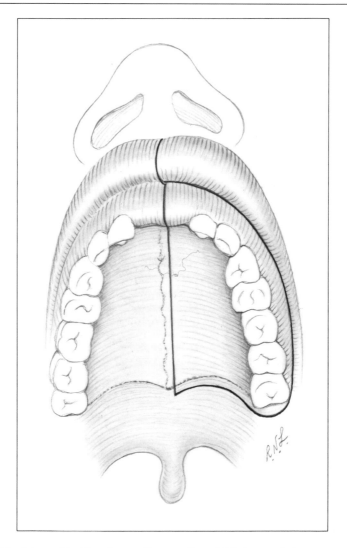

Figure 16.7   Intra-oral incisions for maxillectomy (from RSN, by permission)

4. An incision is made along the orbital rim and the periosteum of the orbit is then elevated superiorly as far as the inferior orbital fissure. This will identify the need for removal of the orbital contents.
5. The maxilla is separated by a series of bony cuts. Figure 16.8 shows the lines of the cuts in the bone, which will be performed with a Stryker saw.
6. The masseter muscle is divided at its attachment and the zygomatic arch is divided. The ethmoidal labyrinth is cleared, allowing the superomedial part of the maxilla to be freed. The hard palate is divided. This can be performed by passing a Gigli saw through the nasal cavity and out between the hard and soft palate, or alternatively a combination of osteotome and chisel can be used.

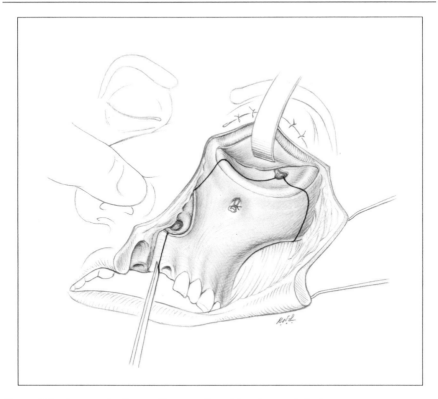

Figure 16.8 Osteotomies for maxillectomy (from RSN, by permission)

7. An osteotome can now be inserted behind the tuberosity of the maxilla and pressure applied in the groove between it and the pterygoid process. Firm pressure may free the posterior wall of the maxilla, although on occasion a sharp blow may be required. This is shown in Figure 16.9. In some instances the maxillary artery may bleed during this procedure. Although this is an uncommon occurrence, if it should occur it is important the specimen is removed quickly and the area packed in the first instance. Once the packing is in place it can then be removed slowly and the maxillary artery ligated.

8. Following the removal of the maxilla it is important also to remove the medial and lateral pterygoid plates to facilitate the fitting of a comfortable prosthesis. Detaching the insertion of temporalis from the mandible is also advisable in controlling post-operative trismus and facilitating a comfortable fit of the prosthesis.

9. The inner surface of the facial skin may be grafted with a split skin graft in order to prevent or reduce facial contraction post-operatively. The wound is closed in two layers. The deep layer is an absorbable suture whereas the skin layer is with a non-absorbable suture such as a 5-0 prolene. The cavity is lightly packed with 2-inch ribbon gauze impregnated with Whiteheads varnish. A temporary prosthesis is laid on to the packing, and wired in place.

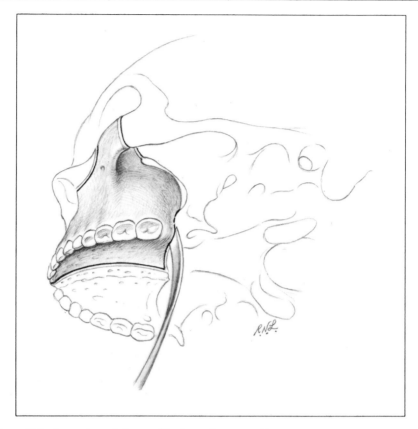

Figure 16.9   Separation of the maxilla from the pterygoid plates with a substantial curved osteotome (from RSN, by permission)

Post-operative care

If the patient has a good fitting prosthesis then a soft diet may be commenced within 1 to 2 days of the surgery. The packing is removed, often under a general anaesthetic, after about 10 days and impressions taken for the permanent prosthesis, which is fitted at 3 weeks.

Chapter 17

Nasal polypectomy and ethmoidectomy

INTRODUCTION

Simple benign nasal polyps are believed to arise in response to a local infective or allergic process in areas of constriction within the nasal cavity, particularly within the ethmoidal air cells and the osteomeatal complex of the paranasal sinuses. Most simple polyps respond to some extent to intra-nasal topical corticosteroids and it is appropriate to use this as first line management. Oral corticosteroids produce more extensive shrinkage of nasal polyps.

If following a reasonable course of intranasal topical corticosteroids (at least 1 to 2 months) the patient is still affected by symptoms such as nasal blockage, a sensation of post-nasal drip/catarrh and anosmia then it is worthwhile removing the nasal polyps. It is not possible to remove every last vestige of nasal polyps surgically, nor is it possible to correct the predisposition to reforming nasal polyps surgically. As a consequence the surgery should be designed to each individual patient whereby the least surgery which effectively relieves the patient's symptoms is appropriate.

Nasal polypectomy is most commonly performed with the use of a headlight although in some centres endoscopic techniques are used. Some surgeons routinely perform an intra-nasal ethmoidectomy at the same time as a nasal polypectomy.

We will describe simple polypectomy, intra-nasal ethmoidectomy and consider endoscopic removal.

SIMPLE NASAL POLYPECTOMY

Indications

The principal indications for removal of nasal polyps are nasal obstruction and a sensation of something running down or hanging down at the back of the nose. Sinusitis as a result of obstructed sinus drainage due to nasal polyps would be an indication for removal.

Any unilateral polyp should be regarded suspiciously and malignancy has to be excluded by urgent removal of the polyp and appropriate histological examination.

Specimen

A nasal polyp is a pedunculated piece of greyish loose and oedematous upper respiratory mucosa. All polyps should be sent for histological examination.

Pre-operative considerations

Simple polyps, especially when solitary, may be removed under topical anaesthesia.

When the polyps are multiple and sessile or when the patient does not wish local anaesthesia, polyps are preferably removed under a general anaesthetic.

Risks

1.   Epistaxis.
2.   Cribriform plate damage and intra-cranial complications.
3.   Damage to the lamina papyracea and orbital complications.
4.   Intra-nasal adhesions.
5.   Failure to remove all of the polyps (particularly those hanging into the nasopharynx) and consequently failure to relieve the patient's symptoms.
6.   Anosmia often persists following nasal polypectomy.

Preparation

The patient should have the nasal lining prepared with a local vasoconstrictive and anaesthetic solution as appropriate.

Patients under local anaesthetic should be in a semi-sitting or reclining position. This has the advantage of preventing the polyps dangling into the nasopharynx such that they are not identified and removed.

If the procedure is to be performed under general anaesthesia then this is delivered through a cuffed peroral endotracheal tube. A throat pack is inserted. The patient is supine on the table with some head-up tilt.

Method

1.   Classically an avulsion snare (a snare in which the wire does not fully retract into the barrel) is insinuated over a polyp and advanced to its base. The snare is closed and then the polyp is gradually removed by gentle avulsion. Figure 17.1 shows the use of a cutting snare in which the snare retracts fully into the barrel and the divided polyp is picked from the nose and removed with Tilly Henckel forceps. A cutting snare should be used for revision surgery.
2.   Alternatively a pair of Tilly Henckel's forceps grasp the base of the polyp and remove it with gentle traction. It is important not to grasp blindly at tissue within the nose. Polyps generally come free with steady traction.
3.   Most simple nasal polyps arise from the ethmoidal air cells and upturned

Citelli's forceps can be used for uncapping the ethmoidal bulla and for removing every visible trace of oedematous mucosa from the air cells. It is important that good visibility is present throughout the procedure.

4. If the surgery has been neat, precise and atraumatic there should be minimal bleeding from the nose and, as such, packing is not required. If bleeding following the polyp removal is particularly persistent then Vaseline gauze packs may be inserted for approximately 12 hours.

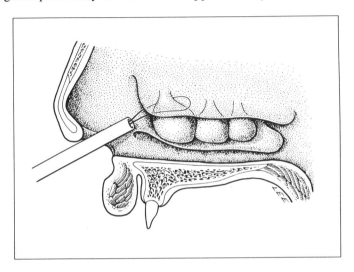

Figure 17.1 The use of a cutting snare to remove nasal polyps from the middle meatus (from RSN, by permission)

Post-operative care

Following general anaesthetic the patient is normally discharged the following day. It is wise to prescribe a regular nasal steroid spray, even following the removal of the polypi, to try to ensure a longer time interval prior to recurrence of the polyps. Mild crusting and blood spotting can occur for 1 to 2 weeks following surgery.

INTRA-NASAL ETHMOIDECTOMY

Indications

Intra-nasal ethmoidectomy is a procedure combined with nasal polypectomy in an attempt to increase the period prior to return of the nasal polyps. Many surgeons believe that in any standard intra-nasal polypectomy a partial ethmoidectomy is performed.

Specimen

Nasal polyps plus bony fragments of the ethmoidal air cells.

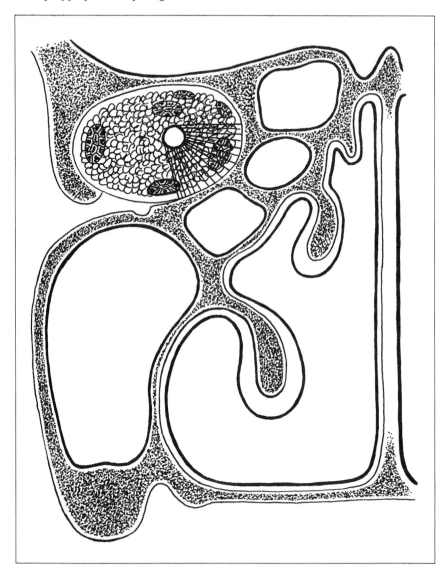

Figure 17.2   Relationship of the ethmoidal air sinuses to the cribriform plate and lamina paparacia

Pre-operative considerations

It is important to realize that the superior part of the ethmoidal air cells lies above the level of the cribriform plate and that the lateral wall of the ethmoidal system is the lamina papyracea which separates the ethmoidal air cells from the orbit.

If instruments penetrate the cribriform plate there is the potential for meningitis or other intra-cranial complications. Penetration of the lamina papyracea risks the development of orbital emphysema or the more serious problems of orbital haematoma and abscess. Figure 17.2 demonstrates these points.

It is crucial that the surgeon undertaking intra-nasal ethmoidectomy should be conversant with the relevant anatomy and should have good visibility during this procedure. Should the operator penetrate too far posteriorly and enter extensively into the posterior ethmoidal air cells, particularly posterior to the posterior ethmoidal artery, then there is a definite risk of damage to the optic nerve.

Risks

1. Bleeding.
2. Failure to remove all of the disease.
3. Orbital emphysema.
4. Orbital haematoma.
5. Orbital abscess.
6. Blindness from:
    -   Damage to the optic nerve.
    -   Orbital haematoma pressing on the nerve.
    -   Thrombophlebitis of orbital veins.
7. Damage to the cribriform plate and consequent intra-cranial complications.

Preparation

The nose is prepared as for nasal polypectomy.

The general anaesthetic is delivered through a cuffed peroral endotracheal tube. A throat pack is inserted. The patient is supine on the table with some head-up tilt. Hypotensive anaesthetic techniques can be of help in reduction of bleeding during this procedure.

Method

1. The nasal polyps are removed in the standard manner. The surgeon then grasps the bases of the polyps and opens the associated air cells around them. Using the Citelli's upturned, straight, or downturned, forceps, as is appropriate to the local anatomy, the air cells are progressively opened from anterior to posterior with the mucosa stripped from the ethmoids. Removal of polypoid tissue is difficult, if not impossible, from the most anterior of the air cells.
2. In general polypoid mucosa separates easily from the air cells with gentle traction. If there is a toughness or a difficulty in removing the polypoid

tissue then one should consider whether it is actually polypoid tissue that is being removed.
3. At the end of the procedure if there is a minimum of bleeding then no packs are required, although if there is still bleeding then the application of Vaseline gauze packs for the next 12 hours is appropriate.

Post-operative care

It is important to check and document the patient's vision immediately he or she recovers from the anaesthetic. Prompt referral to an ophthalmologist is mandatory for any visual disturbance following the surgery. Vision failing post-operatively, after it has been demonstrated to be normal, suggests the development of an intra-orbital thrombophlebitis.

The patient is usually discharged after 24 to 48 hours. It is wise to prescribe a regular nasal steroid spray to try to ensure a longer time interval prior to recurrence of the nasal polyps. Mild crusting and blood spotting can occur for 1 to 2 weeks following surgery.

CLIPPING THE ANTERIOR ETHMOIDAL ARTERY

Indications

1. To reduce bleeding during external ethmoidal sinus surgery.
2. To arrest haemorrhage during endoscopic sinus surgery.
3. To control severe epistaxis of apparent 'ethmoidal' origin.

Pre-operative considerations

The anterior and posterior ethmoidal arteries are branches of the ophthalmic artery within the orbit. They perforate the medial orbital periosteum and transverse the anterior and posterior ethmoidal canals to supply the paranasal sinuses and then return to the cranium prior to entering the nose via the cribriform plate. The anterior ethmoidal artery is approximately 15 mm posterior to the maxillolacrimal suture. It is important to realize that the disposition of the ethmoidal arteries is variable. When the anterior ethmoidal artery is large then the posterior ethmoidal artery is usually small. In a substantial proportion of people the anterior ethmoidal artery may be absent.

Risks

1. Tearing an ethmoidal artery may result in an orbital haematoma. It is wise to involve an ophthalmologist if this occurs. A medial canthotomy may be required to release the tension in the orbit.
2. Orbital damage can result in transient diplopia.
3. Optic nerve damage can occur.

Preparation

General anaesthesia through a peroral endotracheal tube with an oropharyngeal pack in place. A temporary tarsorrhaphy should be performed to avoid risk of damage to the cornea.

Method

1. Figure 14.3A identifies the site of the incision medial to the inner canthus of the eye. The curved 1.5 cm long incision is deepened down to bone. The angular vein may need to be divided. A periosteal elevator is used to deflect progressively the orbital periosteum laterally and dislocate the lacrimal sac out of its groove. A Ferris Smith or similar orbital retractor can be placed within the incision. It is preferable to place the limbs of the Ferris Smith retractor around the anterior ethmoidal artery.
2. Once located, the artery can be occluded either by a ligature or a metal artery clip. Further retraction and progressive posterior periosteal separation will allow location of the posterior ethmoidal artery. The optic nerve can lie between 3 and 7 mm posterior to the posterior ethmoidal artery.
3. The wound is closed with non-absorbable sutures.

Post-operative care

This is usually determined by the reason for ligating the vessels in the first place.

EXTERNAL FRONTAL ETHMOIDECTOMY

Indications

For many years it has been considered that an external approach to the frontal and ethmoidal paranasal sinuses is required when there is extensive disease. The intra-nasal route does not permit adequate access to or visualization of the anterior ethmoid and sphenoid area, nor does it facilitate the identification of reliable landmarks to prevent penetration into the orbit and damage to the cruciform plate.

Extensive disease treated by external frontal ethmoidectomy can be considered to be chronic irreversible mucosal changes in the sinuses, or chronic obstruction to the drainage of the sinuses, or chronic infection.

The procedure described here could be used as an approach to the pituitary fossa and to permit drainage of acute ethmoidal abscesses. Frontal mucocoele can be treated by frontal ethmoidectomy.

Some of the indications for external frontal ethmoidectomy are altering as the development of endoscopic ethmoid surgery proceeds.

Specimen

It is not possible to excise polypoid tissue from a frontal ethmoidectomy en bloc. The specimen is by nature multiple polyps and bony fragments.

Pre-operative considerations

Prior to general anaesthetic the nasal lining should be prepared with a vasoconstrictive solution. Xylometazoline (Otrivine) or its long-acting derivative (Afrazine) is as effective as cocaine solution without the potentially serious complications.

In cases of recurrent purulent infection a prophylactic antibiotic is appropriate. A CT scan of the sinuses should be available to delineate the anatomy.

Risks

1. Orbital haematomas and infections are uncommon.
2. Diplopia and epiphora usually resolve spontaneously within a week of the surgery. Persistent diplopia may require further ophthalmological assessment.
3. Discomfort from the siting of the indwelling tube can often cause problems. Avoidance of the tube impinging on the floor of the nose is important.
4. Damage to the supra-orbital or supratrochlear nerves resulting in anaesthesia of the forehead is not uncommon. Undoubtedly the degree of traction on the upper part of the incision influences this complication.
5. This operation does not always relieve patients of their symptoms.
6. A small depression can appear where the floor of the frontal sinus has been.
7. Intra-cranial complications such as meningitis may occur if there has been damage to the cribriform plate or extensive work within the sphenoid sinus.

Preparation

A general anaesthetic is supplied through a peroral endotracheal tube with a protective throat pack inserted. Hypotensive anaesthetic techniques can be helpful to provide dry operative fields.

The patient lies supine with some foot down tilt of the operating table. The face and forehead should be prepared with a skin preparation which is non-irritant to the eye and conjuctiva. One should never shave the eyebrows. A temporary tarsorrhaphy should be performed to avoid accidental damage to the cornea.

Method

1. A slightly curved incision medial to and concave towards the medial canthus of the eye is used. This incision is extended upwards and laterally

to permit access to the frontal sinus. Care should be taken to avoid damage to the trochlea of the superior oblique muscle. Figure 14.3A shows the basic position of the incision. The incision is deepened through the periosteum and onto bone. The angular vein occasionally has to be ligated.

2. Subperiosteal elevation should reveal the nasal process of both the maxilla and the frontal bone and the medial orbital wall. The lacrimal sac is elevated from its groove and displaced laterally. The subperiosteal dissection continues posteriorly along the lamina papyracea to identify the ethmoidal vessels as the exit from the orbital cavity. A Ferris Smith retractor is inserted, which facilitates the isolation of the ethmoidal vessels, which are ligated with sutures or with clips and then divided.

3. Figure 17.3 demonstrates the exposure into the ethmoidal air cells with a Ferris Smith retractor in place. The ethmoidal air cells are entered and progressively exenterated to identify the insertion of the middle and superior turbinates. The cribriform plate should be identified superiorly and the ostium into the sphenoidal sinuses identified posteriorly. Visualization of the ethmoidal sinuses through the nose can often be of help to ensure removal of all the ethmoidal air cells.

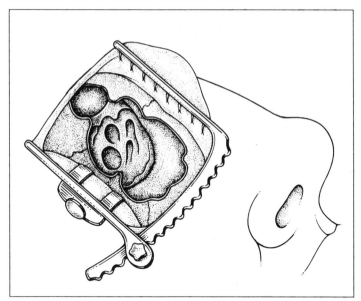

Figure 17.3 Exposure of the middle ethmoidal air cells and frontal sinus floor (from RSN, by permission)

4. It is safest to penetrate the anterior wall of the sphenoid sinus at its inferomedial part. It is then possible to open the anterior wall of the sinus progressively and avoid damage to any structures lateral to the sinus which are at risk, particularly if the sinus walls are deficient.

5. To open into the frontal sinus one should continue upwards through the anterior ethmoidal cells until the floor of the frontal sinus is exposed. The mid-line septa of the frontal sinus can be a long way from the mid-line and it is worth reviewing the radiographs to ensure that the correct sinus is entered. With punch forceps the channel from the ethmoidal to the frontal

sinus is widened and the diseased contents of the frontal sinus evacuated. The use of a large burr and drill to smooth down all sharp points of bone in this area can be very helpful.

6. With exenteration of the frontal and ethmoidal air cells it is now important to maintain continuity between the frontal sinus and the nose. A wide bore tube is inserted which extends from the frontal sinus to the nasal cavity. Portex tubing, as used in endotracheal anaesthetic tubes, is very suitable. The tube is left in place usually for 2 to 3 months. If there is any doubt as to the ability to retain the tube then it can be suture anchored to the surrounding bone.
7. Vaseline gauze impregnated with bismuth iodoform paraffin paste (BIPP) is inserted into the nasal cavity if there is persistent bleeding, although if there is a minimum of bleeding then no packing is required.
8. The wound is closed in two layers with 3-0 chromic catgut to the deep layer and 5-0 prolene to the skin. The cutaneous sutures can be removed after 5 days.

Post-operative care

Any packing is removed after 24 to 48 hours. Antibiotics are usually continued for about 5 days after the operation. It is helpful to suck out the indwelling tube regularly after the procedure. The end of the frontal sinus tube should not be allowed to impinge on to the floor of the nose as this may result in granulation tissue formation and discomfort for the patient. If there is a danger of this happening the tube should be shortened. The tube is removed after 3 months.

Transient diplopia and occasional epiphora follow this procedure and generally settle within a few days.

ENDOSCOPIC ETHMOIDECTOMY AND FRONTAL RECESS EXPLORATION

Indications

The indications for endoscopic ethmoidectomy and frontal recess exploration are still being defined. The indications, however, may include:

1. Polypoid sinusitis.
2. Nasal obstruction/congestion at the bridge of the nose.
3. Recurrent facial pain due to osteomeatal complex or ethmoidal sinus disease.
4. Mucocoeles of the ethmoidal complex, the frontal sinus or the maxillary sinus.
5. Retention cysts of the maxillary sinus.
6. Recurrent maxillary sinusitis due to obstruction of the osteomeatal complex.
7. Post-nasal drip.

8. Mycotic sinusitis.
9. Antrochoanal polyps.
10. Persistent problems and complaints after open sinus operations.

Specimen

Nasal polyps and bony fragments.

Pre-operative considerations

Prior to performing functional endoscopic sinus surgery the operator should be fully conversant with the relevant anatomy. Cadaver dissections plus attendance at an endoscopic sinus surgery course are probably essential.

Coronal CT scans with 4 mm cuts are required prior to this form of surgery. The scans permit identification of disease and provide an anatomical map to prevent avoidable complications. The scans should be available at the time of operation.

An endoscopic examination of the nose before surgery is required, both to identify the presence of disease within the middle meatus and to determine whether the surgery is technically possible without first correcting, for example, a septal deformity.

Risks

1. Blindness from damage to the optic nerve.
2. Intra-orbital bleeding. Urgent ophthalmological consultation and a lateral canthotomy may be required in this situation.
3. Laceration of the internal carotid artery (this is related to posterior ethmoidal surgery).
4. Cerebral spinal fluid leak (meningitis risk).
5. Synechia or adhesions within the middle meatus.
6. Bleeding. If the surgeon's view is obscured by an excess of blood then the procedure should be abandoned.
7. Orbital emphysema as a result of breaching the lamina papyracea. The patient should be advised not to blow the nose following this form of surgery in an effort to avoid this complication.
8. Failure to relieve the symptoms. This most commonly occurs when there has been a failure to remove all of the disease.
9. Increased post-nasal drip is common post-operatively for approximately 3–4 weeks.

Preparation

This form of surgery should be performed under local anaesthesia with sedation. This technique of anaesthesia orbital complications. General anaesthesia can, on occasion, be used by the experienced operator. In this circumstance the endoscopic procedure should be limited to an uncinectomy, middle meatal antrostomy and opening of the ethmoidal bulla. Extensive surgery under general anaesthesia carries considerable risk.

The patient has xylometazoline (Otrivine) sprayed into the nose prior to transfer to the operating room. The surgeon prepares ribbon gauze soaked in cocaine 10% solution and inserts these lightly as packs into each nostril. The surgeon injects lignocaine 1% with 1:200 000 adrenaline into the lateral wall of the middle meatus over the uncinate process. Figure 17.4 demonstrates the points of injection.

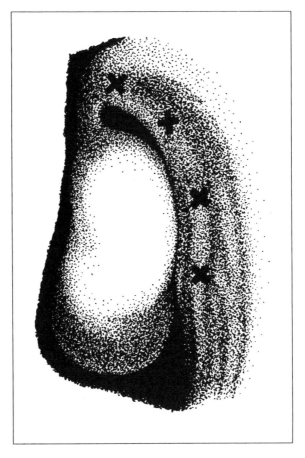

Figure 17.4   Injection points in the lateral wall of the nose prior to uncinectomy. The middle turbinate and middle meatus are illustrated

It is preferable to have an anaesthetist present during functional endoscopic sinus surgery. An indwelling Venflon is preferable. The patient should be monitored with ECG and a pulse oximeter. An individual anaesthetist may choose a combination of narcotic or benzodiazepine drugs to produce sedation.

Oxygen can be given through nasal prongs attached to the mouth. The patient should be in a state such that he or she can answer questions should the surgeon ask them.

The patient is laid supine on the table, which is tilted foot-down.

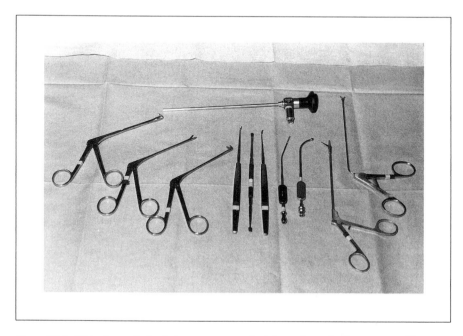

Figure 17.5 This shows the basic instruments required for endoscopic sinus surgery. The tapes around the shafts of these instruments are in different colours. The operating assistant has an index for the names of these instruments related to their coloured tapes. This simplifies handing the surgeon the correct instrument

Method

1. Surgery is performed with the 0 degree forward looking 4 mm telescope. The surgeon commences by removing the uncinate process. A sickle knife is used, kept in a plane parallel to the lateral wall of the nose, to incise the uncinate process from superior to inferior. A Freer's elevator is used to reflect the uncinate process medially. The uncinate is then grasped in a pair of fine Tilly Henckel's forceps and removed.

2. The opening into the maxillary antrum is at the root of uncinate process at the superior margin of the inferior turbinate. Figure 17.5 shows the basic instruments for functional endoscopic sinus surgery. Any polypoid disease is removed from the osteomeatal complex and then the maxillary opening can be enlarged. This can be done either posteriorly or anteriorly. A small pair of backward biting forceps (Ostrum's) are useful for this procedure.

3. At the apex of where the uncinate has been removed is the entrance into the frontal recess. Figure 17.6 shows this. A pair of forceps can be insinuated into the frontal recess and closed. This allows polypoid tissue to be

removed from the frontal recess. When treating a frontal mucocoele this procedure is often followed by a release of mucopus.

4. The safe place to open the ethmoidal bulla is in the inferomedial face of the bulla. Once opened, any polypoid tissue is removed. Although it is important to remove the polypoid disease it is not essential to break down all the septa of the ethmoidal air cells (Figure 17.7).

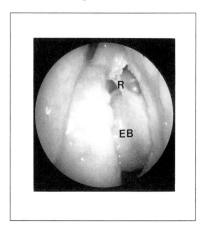

Figure 17.6 Exposure of the frontal recess after removal of the uncinate process. (R) marks the frontal recess. (EB) marks the ethmoidal bulla

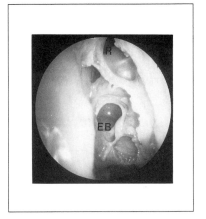

Figure 17.7 The ethmoidal bulla has been opened. The frontal process is shown superiorly. (R) marks the frontal recess. (EB) marks the ethmoidal bulla

5. The posterior wall of the ethmoidal bulla (also called the basal lamella or the ground lamella) is the anterior wall of the posterior ethmoidal air cells. The optic nerve lies posterolateral to the posterior ethmoidal air cells. Penetration of the posterior wall of the ethmoidal bulla brings the surgeon into the area of risk to the optic nerve.

6. In those few cases, in which one has to enter the posterior ethmoidal cells, the initial puncture should be performed at the inferomedial part of the basal lamella. The operator can then enlarge progressively laterally. Reference to appropriate coronal CT scans is required during this part of the operation.

7. Depending on the extent and nature of surgery, plus the amount of damage to the lateral surface of the middle turbinate, the patient may be left without any nasal packs, with a thin strip of ribbon gauze in the middle meatus, with a small Mercel sponge or with a small silastic sheet inserted.

Post-operative care

Gauze strips are removed after 3–6 hours. Mercel sponges are removed after 48 hours and splints after 5–10 days. The nose is aspirated the day after surgery and the patient reviewed after one week. It is important when the middle meatus is open that routine and regular aspiration is performed to prevent collection of crusts within the meatus.

In cases of polypoid disease then topical intranasal steroids, such as Betnesol aqueous drops or Beconase nasal spray, should be commenced in the post-operative period to prevent further recurrence of disease.

Chapter 18

Surgery of the frontal sinus

INTRODUCTION

In the last few years the indications for surgery to the frontal sinus have reduced. The development of endoscopic sinus surgery may further reduce the need for external frontal sinus operations. Mucocoeles or pyocoeles of the frontal sinus may be adequately treated by a frontal recess endoscopic approach and this is a useful procedure prior to performing an external trephine. The external frontal-ethmoidectomy is discussed on page 213 of Chapter 17 on ethmoidectomy, while endoscopic ethmoidectomy is discussed on page 216 of Chapter 17.

In this chapter we will consider the procedure of external frontal sinus drainage and the bifrontal osteoplastic flap.

FRONTAL SINUS TREPHINE

Indications

Trephining the frontal sinus is required for the acutely obstructed frontal sinus in which frontal sinus pain and extreme tenderness persist, despite adequate treatment with intravenous antibiotics and nasal decongestants. When the skills are available an initial endoscopic procedure should be attempted. In general, failure to relieve severe symptoms after 24–48 hours of medical therapy is an indication for trephine surgery.

Complications outwith the frontal sinus are also an indication for surgery. Examples of these would be the development of a subperiosteal abscess or intracranial complication.

Specimen

Pus for culture and sensitivity.

Pre-operative considerations

Plain sinus radiographs should be available prior to the operation. They can be helpful in identifying the anatomy of the sinuses. A CT scan will provide superior relevant anatomical information.

Risks

Complications specific to the trephine of the frontal sinus are unusual, but complications of the disease itself can be both insidious and dangerous. Examples of such complications include:

1. Osteomyelitis of the frontal bone.
2. Intracranial venous thrombophlebitis.
3. Extradural abscess.
4. Meningitis.
5. Subdural abscess.
6. Brain abscess.

Preparation

General anaesthesia delivered through an oral endotracheal tube with a protective throat pack in place. The patient is supine on the table with a foot-down tilt. The skin, upper face and forehead are prepared with a solution which is harmless to the eyes. A temporary tarsorrhaphy is performed to avoid accidental corneal damage.

Method

1. The incision is placed parallel and medial to the normal position of the eyebrow. The incision is deepened through the skin, subcutaneous tissue and periosteum. Bipolar diathermy can be very helpful in controlling bleeding. Figure 18.1 demonstrates the site of incision.
2. The periosteum is stripped from the floor of the frontal sinus. The floor can be perforated using either a drill and burr or a small gouge and hammer. Typically there is a release of pus under pressure when the true frontal sinus is entered. A swab is taken for bacteriological culture.
3. If there is an absence of pus this may mean that a frontal ethmoidal cell has been opened. A careful removal of the roof of this cell will lead into the true frontal sinus, resulting in drainage. Plain radiographs or a CT scan may warn of this possibility.
4. The posterosuperior walls of the sinus should be thoroughly inspected and if clinically indicated then a portion of the roof of the sinus may have to be removed to identify and drain an extradural abscess.
5. A small drainage tube should be inserted into the sinus at the end of the operation and secured with a stitch.

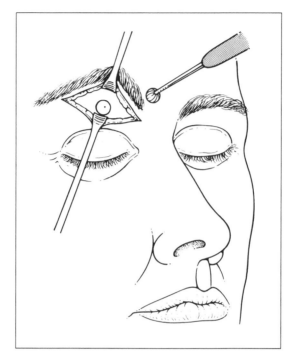

Figure 18.1   Exposure of the site for frontal sinus trephine (from RSN, by permission)

Post-operative care

The sinus should be washed out through the indwelling tube, for a period of about 48 hours. Nasal decongestant therapy should be continued and appropriate antibiotic therapy, which may be modified depending on the results of bacteriological culture, continued for 7–10 days. Infection in the other paranasal sinuses should be treated.

OSTEOPLASTIC FRONTAL FLAP OPERATION

Indications

This approach can be used to remove a frontal osteoma, remove a mucocoele, explore the posterior wall of the frontal sinus or alternatively to remove chronically infected mucosa. The development of endoscopic sinus surgery by altering the management of frontal mucocoele and 'chronic sinusitis' may reduce the need for the osteoplastic flap procedure.

Pre-operative considerations

Prior to the operation a plain fronto-occipital radiograph should be taken while the patient has two crossed wires taped to the forehead. This radiograph accompanies the patient to the operating room. The frontal sinus outline is cut out with scissors to form a template. Once the patient is anaesthetized the template is superimposed on the wires on the forehead and the outline of the sinus can then be tattooed on the skin through the periosteum with methylene blue. This is shown in Figure 18.2.

Those patients in whom a bitemporal coronal incision is planned should wash their hair in a chlorhexidine or similar shampoo daily for 3 days prior to the operation.

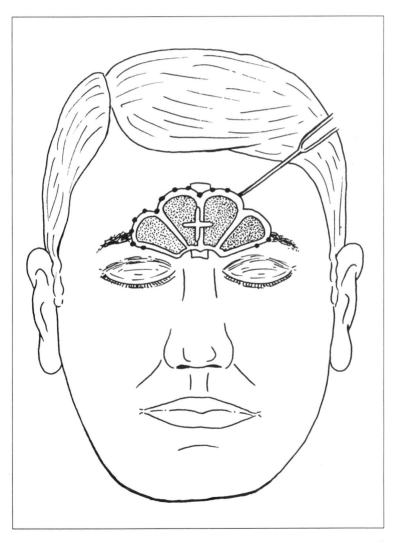

Figure 18.2   This shows the tattooing of the methylene blue over the template to outline the frontal sinus

Risks

1. Haematoma.
2. Forehead anaesthesia. The eyebrow incision almost invariably divides supraorbital and supratrochleal nerve, resulting in forehead anaesthesia. These nerves, however, can also be damaged inadvertently during the bitemporal flap.
3. Nasal discomfort from the indwelling tube.
4. Infection in the sinus and osteomyelitis arising either from failure to eradicate chronically infected tissue within the sinus or avascular necrosis of the fat within the frontal sinus. This is a potentially serious complication as it may lead to intracranial problems. If there is any doubt, parenteral antibiotics are indicated. It is worth remembering that radiological changes of infection may take 4–6 weeks to develop.

Preparation

General anaesthesia delivered through an oral endotracheal anaesthesia with a protective throat pack. The patient is supine on the table, which is tilted foot-down. Temporary tarsorrhaphies to both eyes help protect the corneas from abrasion.

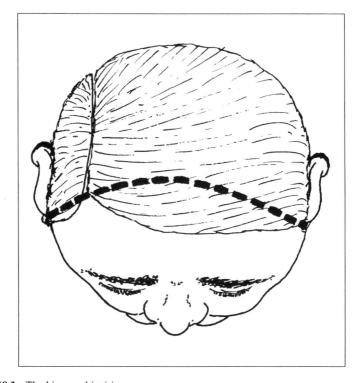

Figure 18.3 The bicoronal incision

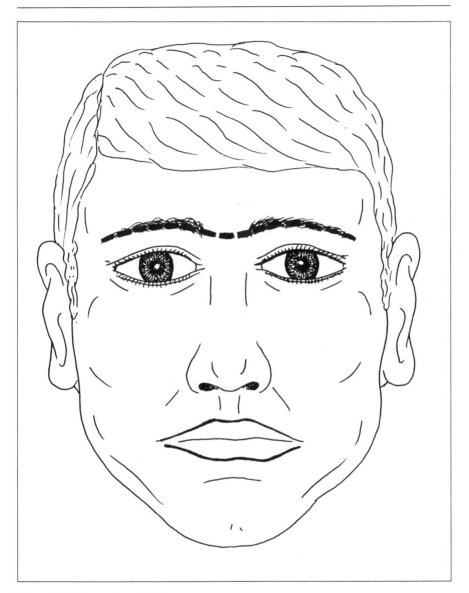

Figure 18.4 The eyebrow incision

Method

1. The bitemporal coronal incision is performed immediately anterior to the interaural coronal line as shown in Figure 18.3. As the cranial cavity is not entered hair does not need to be removed. The incision is deepened through the aponeurosis and the flap elevated forwards to the supraorbital ridges. Raney clips are placed on the flap edges to ensure haemostasis.

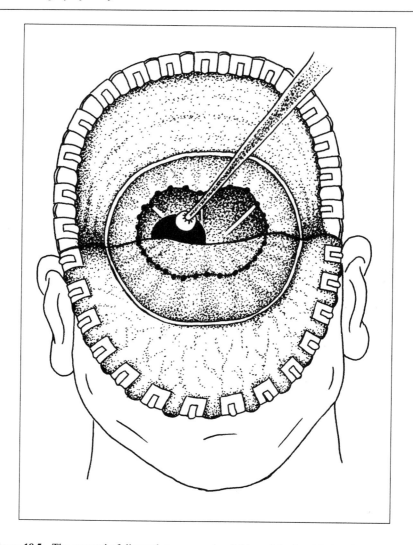

Figure 18.5   The removal of diseased mucosa and polishing of the frontal sinus bone

2. If there is a strong family history of baldness or the patient is bald then an eyebrow incision which runs through both eyebrows and connects across the mid-line can be used as in Figure 18.4. The eyebrows are not shaved. This incision almost invariably produces forehead anaesthesia.
3. The periosteum is incised approximately 2.5 cm outside the tattoo marks. This periosteum is elevated to inside the tattoo marks. A Stryker saw is used to outline the bone flap, which is then elevated free with the use of osteotomes. This is shown in Figure 18.5. With the bone free an osteoma can be excised, diseased mucosa removed and the posterior sinus wall inspected.

4. The sinus can now either be obliterated with fat obtained from the abdominal cavity or the operator should open the frontal recess and ethmoidal air cells to create a large passage into the nose. If a large passage is created into the nose then a portex tube should be sited, as described in the section on external frontal ethmoidectomy, page 216, Chapter 17.
5. The bone flap is returned and the periosteum sutured with chromic catgut. A suction drain is inserted. The wound is closed in two layers with a deep absorbable layer and non-absorbable sutures or clips to skin.

Post-operative care

If there has been infection within the sinus or if the sinus has been obliterated with fat then post-operative antibiotic cover is appropriate. The drains should be removed when there is minimal drainage. Those patients who have a portex tube in place should have regular after-care to ensure that this tube does not become blocked and that it is removed after about 3 to 4 months.

Chapter 19

Endoscopy of the upper aerodigestive tracts

Endoscopy is the visual examination of a body cavity, hollow viscus or space through a specifically designed instrument. The endoscope is basically a tube with an optical and a lighting system. In otolaryngology there are three principal forms of endoscopy:

1. Fibre-optic flexible endoscopy.
2. Hopkin's rod rigid telescope endoscopy.
3. Direct (rigid) endoscopy.

Fibre-optic endoscopy involves a device in which a bundle of fibre-optic strands are collected together into a flexible instrument which has the ability to be manipulated 'round corners'. The illumination runs through some of the fibre-optic threads and the operator receives a 'picture' from the distal end of the endoscope through other fibre-optic bundles which constitute the endoscope. The fibre-optic endoscope has been designed into a number of diameters and lengths. Pernasal examination of the post-nasal space, the pharynx and larynx can be performed with short and thin fibre-optic endoscopes. Typically these endoscopes have diameters less than 5 mm and lengths of approximately 300 mm.

Small fibre-optic endoscopes do not have associated channels through which irrigation, suction and biopsy forceps can be applied. As the size of the endoscopes increases, however, these features are incorporated and they are typically found in fibre-optic bronchoscopes and oesophagogastroscopes.

FIBRE-OPTIC LARYNGOSCOPY

Introduction

Diagnostic pernasal fibre-optic laryngoscopy is a common out-patient diagnostic procedure.

Indications

1. Pernasal fibre-optic laryngoscopy is indicated in the assessment of laryngo-

pharyngeal pathology whenever indirect laryngoscopy by mirror is inadequate.
2. A thin fibre-optic laryngoscope (3 mm diameter) can be of use in the assessment of neonatal congenital stridor without recourse to general anaesthetic.

Pre-operative considerations

Fibre-optic endoscopy does not replace indirect laryngoscopy by mirror examination. Mirror examination provides a superior view of the base of the tongue, vallecula and anterior surface of the epiglottis. These areas are not well seen by fibre-optic endoscopy. It is often difficult to demonstrate the anterior commissure of the larynx on mirror examination and in this area the fibre-optic instrument performs well. The bases of the pyriform fossae and the post-cricoid region are not seen on either mirror or pernasal fibre-optic laryngoscopy. These areas require direct endoscopic assessment.

Preparation

The patient is sat in a chair and has the procedure explained. The side of the nose with the clearer passage is prepared with topical anaesthetic. In those patients with a particularly active gag reflex the oropharynx may also be sprayed with topical anaesthetic.

Method

1. The examiner checks the controls of the endoscope, lightly smears the shaft of the endoscope with lubricant and applies a demister to the tip of the endoscope. The demister may be an alcohol swab, warm water or a disinfectant solution.
2. Figure 19.1 shows pernasal fibre-optic laryngoscopy commencing. The examiner should advance the instrument tip under direct vision using manipulation of the endoscopic tip as the means to curve through the nasopharynx. Parts of the nasal cavity, the Eustachian tubes and the nasopharynx can be assessed with the fibre-optic endoscope, although the rigid Hopkin's rod nasal telescopes are better tools for this task. The competence of nasopharyngeal closure can be viewed by asking the patient to phonate and swallow while the tip of the endoscope is in the nasopharynx.
3. The tip of the endoscope is advanced into the pharynx and past the upper border of the epiglottis to view the larynx. The examiner should systematically view the structures of the pharynx, larynx and closure of the vocal cords on phonation.
4. Occasionally mucus can obstruct the endoscopic view as the instrument is advanced past the base of the tongue. In this situation either retract the endoscope until a view appears or ask the patient to swallow. The swallow may wipe the mucus clear from the endoscopic tip.

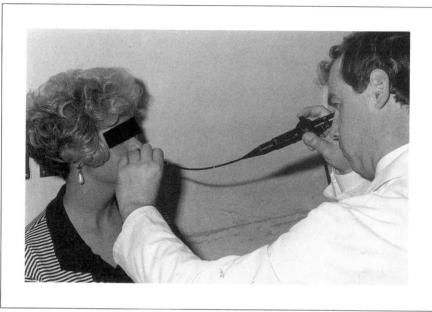

Figure 19.1   This shows the initial insertion of a fibre-optic flexible nasal endoscope

FIBRE-OPTIC BRONCHOSCOPY (PERNASAL)

Introduction

The fibre-optic bronchoscope has a wider diameter and a greater length than the fibre-optic laryngoscope. The instrument usually contains both an aspiration/insufflation channel and a channel for biopsy forceps.

Indications

1. The diagnostic evaluation of the trachea and the bronchial tree up to the third and fourth divisions.
2. The evaluation of haemoptysis.
3. To remove obstructing bronchial plugs of mucus following a general anaesthetic or in ventilated patients.
4. The diagnosis of peripheral lung lesions when transbronchial biopsy is performed under radiographic control.

Pre-operative considerations

Fibre-optic bronchoscopy is useful in those patients with marked kyphosis or severe arthritis of the cervical spine. Rigid bronchoscopy is preferable for foreign body removal or in the assessment of a vascular tumour when it is possible to pack onto the lesion in cases of haemorrhage.

A thorough knowledge of bronchial anatomy is mandatory prior to performing either flexible or rigid bronchoscopy (Figure 19.2).

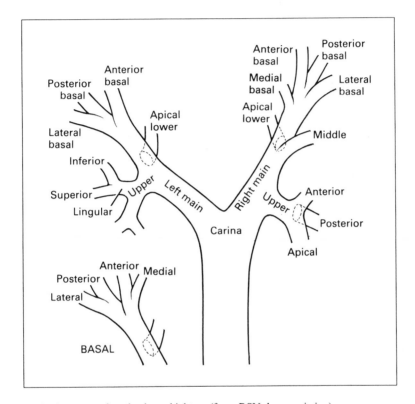

Figure 19.2 Anatomy of tracheobronchial tree (from RSN, by permission)

Risks

Flexible fibre-optic bronchoscopy is a safe procedure where complications are unusual. Risks include:

1. Bleeding following biopsy.
2. Local anaesthetic reaction.
3. Oxygen desaturation.
4. Pneumothorax (rare).

Preparation

The nose, pharynx and larynx are prepared with topical anaesthetic. Oxygen insufflated through a catheter can be used in those patients with obstructive airways disease. The patient is semi-recumbent.

Method

1. The examiner, standing to the right and facing the patient, passes the fibre-optic bronchoscope through the wider nasal passage.
2. When the tip of the instrument is immediately proximal to the vocal cords a small quantity of topical local anaesthetic such as lignocaine 4% is instilled through the broncoscope on to the cords and through the glottis. After 2 minutes the fibre-optic instrument can be advanced into the trachea. As the examination proceeds, further instillations of topical anaesthetic are required to anaesthetize the trachea and bronchi.
3. The tracheobronchial examination should proceed systematically and it is crucial to remember that the position of the tip of the scope can only be calculated by reference to landmarks already negotiated.
4. Brush biopsies, direct biopsies and aspirates can be obtained through the flexible fibre-optic bronchoscope although one should remember that the forceps can often not be withdrawn when the tip of the instrument is deflected.

FIBRE-OPTIC OESOPHAGOGASTROSCOPY

Fibre-optic oesophagogastroscopy is generally performed by a medical or surgical gastroenterologist. The endoscope is passed through the mouth in a patient who is mildly sedated. A guard should always be worn by those patients who have teeth, to avoid the patient biting and damaging the endoscope. This endoscope is excellent in the evaluation of the digestive tract beyond the post-cricoid region. Even with the technique of careful retraction of the oesophago-gastroscope through the cricopharyngeus, pharynx and larynx this instrument does not permit satisfactory evaluation of these areas. Rigid endoscopy is required to 'open up' and fully assess the pyriform fossae and the post-cricoid region of the oesophagus.

In general, foreign bodies should not be removed from the oesophagus with a flexible oesophagogastroscope. Rigid oesophagoscopes facilitate the use of strong forceps and permit the simple retraction of sharp foreign bodies either into or through the beak of the endoscope. This prevents a trailing sharp point from ripping the oesophageal lining as the endoscope is removed.

HOPKIN'S ROD RIGID TELESCOPE ENDOSCOPY

These rigid instruments contain a glass rod lens system (Hopkin's system) which is superior to the traditional multiple small lens optical system. The Hopkin's system permits a smaller diameter of instrument, a larger viewing angle and a brighter image compared with the older system. These points have facilitated the introduction of these telescopes into otolaryngology.

These telescopes can have deflection angles (viewing angles) of 0°, 30°, 70°, 90° or 120°.

There are a different number of lengths and diameters of these endoscopes. These telescopes can be passed through a rigid endoscope to provide a 'close-up' or angled view of a region or lesion. For example, at direct laryngoscopy the 90° telescope gives a superior view of the subglottis.

The 90° telescope can be used through the mouth to examine the post-nasal space.

RIGID NASAL ENDOSCOPY

The adult nasal telescopes are 18 cm long with an outer diameter of 4.0 mm. The endoscopes of 0° and 30° deflection are the most useful. It is possible with these instruments to examine the nasal cavity thoroughly and to assess the nasopharynx and the medial ends of the Eustachian tubes.

Preparation

The patient is sat semi-recumbent. A topical anaesthetic and vasoconstrictive spray are applied to the nasal lining. Useful information on the nasal cavity is gained if the operator examines the nose with a headlight while applying the topical spray. The end of the endoscope is demisted with an alcohol swab or disinfectant solution.

Method

The instrument tip is inserted past the nasal vestibule before the operator looks through the eye piece. Figure 19.3 shows the commencement of endoscopic examination. For an initial assessment the 30° endoscope is ideal and the examiner should systematically view the floor of the nose, the inferior meatus and turbinate, the middle meatus and turbinate, the superior meatus and turbinate, the olfactory cleft and the nasal septum. The endoscope tip is then passed along the floor of the nose into the nasopharynx and by rotating the instrument the entire nasopharynx can be assessed.

To perform endoscopic nasal surgery the 0° endoscope is appropriate. Functional endoscopic sinus surgery is covered in the section on ethmoidal sinus surgery, Chapter 17, page 216.

RIGID ENDOSCOPY: DIRECT LARYNGOSCOPY

Indications

1. Direct laryngoscopy is required to diagnose a lesion within the larynx which cannot be dealt with by indirect or fibre-optic laryngoscopy.

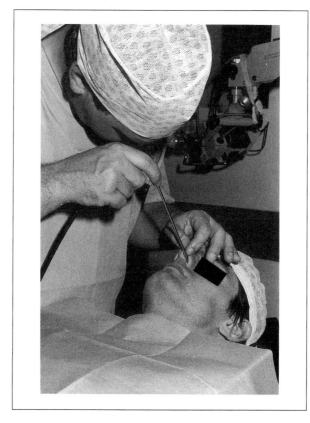

Figure 19.3 The surgeon opens the nasal vestibule by everting the nasal tip, with a finger, at the same time as inserting the rigid nasal telescope

2. Direct laryngoscopy allows tissue to be removed for histological analysis.
3. Foreign bodies can be removed and lesions of the larynx treated through the laryngoscope.
4. The mobility of the cricoarytenoid joints can be assessed by palpation.
5. The microscope can be added to a suspended laryngoscope (see later in this section) for more precise work within the larynx. A CO_2 laser can be added to the microscope to allow precise treatment of interlaryngeal lesions.
6. Teflon or similar material can be injected lateral to the vocal cord in the treatment of the unilateral vocal cord paralysis.

Specimen

This will depend precisely on the lesion being treated. It is always very important when 'biopsying' potentially malignant tumours of the pharynx and larynx that very careful labelling is made of the various points from which suspicious lesions are removed and that an accurate post-operative record and illustration are made.

Pre-operative considerations

1. The state of the patient's dentition and the presence of expensive dental crowns should be assessed. The patient should be warned prior to surgery that there is always a risk of damage to teeth or crowns during the performance of rigid endoscopy.
2. The mobility of the neck should be checked and where there is any doubt as to the mobility of the cervical spine then a lateral soft tissue X-ray of the neck should be obtained. This is often of greater importance for rigid oesophagoscopy.
3. When the laryngoscopy is being performed for assessment of a malignant tumour one should consider whether airway obstruction may occur either at the time of intubation or in the post-operative period and warn the patient that a tracheostomy may be placed at the time of surgery should an airway problem develop. In those patients in whom the airway is perilous an initial tracheostomy under local anaesthetic prior to direct laryngoscopy is preferable to a failed intubation by the anaesthetist.
4. As the surgeon and the anaesthetist are competing for the same space during a direct laryngoscopy it is important that there is close co-operation and liaison prior to the operation.

Risks

1. Dental damage.
2. Abrasion to the upper alveolus in the edentulous patient.
3. Damage to the lips from instrument manipulation.

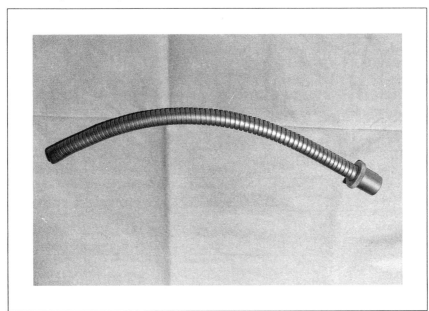

Figure 19.4   The flexible Oswal Hunton laser anaesthetic tube

4. Haematoma formation over the posterior pharyngeal wall.
5. Laryngeal obstruction from swelling following surgery.
6. Failure to get sufficient tissue for histological diagnosis.
7. Anterior commissure webbing as a result of extensive manipulation or surgery at the anterior commissure.
8. Pulmonary complications from inhaled blood or debris.

Preparation

1. A general anaesthetic delivered through a small bore endotracheal tube is usually appropriate. There are a number of different tubes and catheters through which to deliver the anaesthetic agents and undoubtedly individual anaesthetists will have their preference. As a surgeon the preference should be for the smallest bore tube and the technique with which the anaesthetist is happy.
2. If a laser is to be used then a metal tube, such as the Oswal Hunton tube (Figure 19.4), will be required. The lower respiratory tract has to be protected by wet cottonoid swabs from accidental laser strikes and the anaesthetist should use the least inflammable anaesthetic gases. The patient must be protected thoroughly from accidental laser strikes by being covered with wet towels. A warning notice must go on the door to theatre to show that a laser is in action and the members of staff within the operating room need to wear protective goggles to prevent accidental laser strikes of their eyes.
3. In some circumstances, such as Teflon injection to the vocal cords, local anaesthetic is preferable. This requires close co-operation between the anaesthetist and the surgeon. Typically cocaine swabs are held within the pyriform fossa with appropriately designed forceps. The anaesthetist often uses a sedative agent during the procedure and may have arranged to have oxygen insufflated through the laryngoscope once it is in place. The advantage of this technique for Teflon injection of the vocal cord is that it allows the voice to be assessed and the quantity of injected Teflon to be titrated against the voice.
4. The surgeon should confirm the correct scopes, light cables and instruments for endolaryngeal surgery are available prior to commencing the procedure.
5. The patient is placed supine on the table and the head is extended on the atlas with the neck flexed. This position is often called 'sniffing the morning air'. It can be achieved by placing a pillow partly under the shoulders and partly under the head of the patient. Plumping the pillow allows the ideal position to be achieved. Alternatively, a head rest and sandbag can be used to achieve the same result. One technique is shown in Figure 2.1 (p. 13).

Method

1. A shield is inserted to protect the teeth. If the patient is edentulous a gauze swab or gum shield should be laid over the upper alveolus to prevent abrasion during the endoscopy.

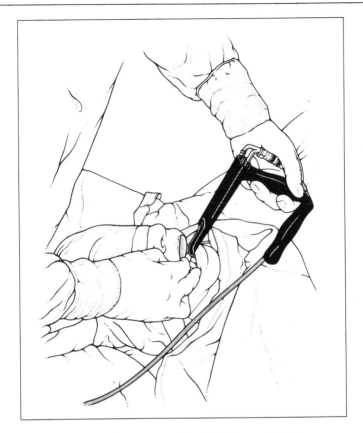

Figure 19.5 Insertion of a rigid laryngoscope (from RSN, by permission)

2. Figure 19.5 shows the initial position for insertion of the laryngoscope. The surgeon stands and opens the mouth with his or her free hand. The laryngoscope is placed on the tongue and the uvula identified. Downward pressure on the tongue opens the mouth and often an excess of saliva requires to be aspirated at this point. The surgeon identifies the uvula and slowly inserts the laryngoscope over the base of the tongue.

3. The second landmark to be identified is the tip of the epiglottis. At this point the surgeon usually sits down and then lifts the tip of the epiglottis upwards and advances the scope till the larynx comes into view, as in Figure 19.6. Sometimes it can be useful to follow the endotracheal tube into the larynx. The endotracheal tube should be sitting between the posterior glottis.

4. If the laryngoscopy is being performed to assess a potentially malignant lesion within the larynx then it is important to assess all other parts of the pharynx and larynx prior to performing a biopsy. In this way the surgeon will avoid blood contaminating his or her field and obscuring the second or contiguous part of the lesion. The surgeon should mentally go through a checklist of all the areas within the pharynx and larynx that he or she is deliberately viewing prior to assessment of the laryngeal lesion. In some circumstances this may necessitate a change of scope. An oesophagoscope

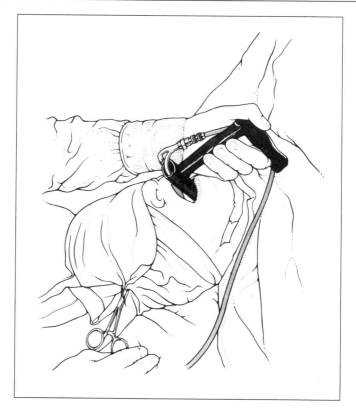

Figure 19.6 Advancing the laryngoscope into the larynx (from RSN, by permission)

may be required to assess the post-cricoid and upper oesophagus, whereas the anterior commissure scope may be required to assess the subglottis, the anterior commissure and on occasion the laryngeal ventricles.

5. One sequence of observation would be first to look at the vallecula on each side, to inspect the lateral and posterior pharyngeal wall, to inspect the laryngeal surface of the epiglottis, to examine each pyriform fossa in turn and to follow the aryepiglottic fold to the posterior part of the larynx, to inspect the post-cricoid and upper oesophageal ventricles and the anterior commissure, plus an inspection of the subglottis. A rigid bronchoscopy may be performed at the same time.

6. When a patient is being assessed for a malignant lesion of the larynx or pharynx the opportunity should always be taken, with a patient under general anaesthetic, to examine the neck thoroughly and so identify any lymphadenopathy.

7. Following the completion of examination of other areas of the pharynx, oesophagus and larynx then a biopsy or appropriate surgery of the laryngeal lesion is performed through the laryngoscope.

Microlaryngoscopy

In some circumstances the surgeon now proceeds to microlaryngoscopy. The magnification and the ability for the surgeon to use two hands greatly facilitates delicate procedures within the laryngeal cavity.

1. A purpose-built table is placed over the chest of the patient and 400 mm objective lens is inserted in to the microscope.
2. There is a specifically designed set of endoscopes and instruments for microlaryngoscopy produced by Kleinsasser, who pioneered the technique. The scopes are black with a matt finish to prevent reflection. These scopes are held by a clamp attached by a ratchet to the chest piece, which allows the surgeon's hands to be released for dissection. A variety of angled forceps, scissors and suckers are available for the surgery. Figure 19.7 shows the attachment of the clamp and ratchet to the laryngoscope. The surgeon keeps a close eye on the laryngeal glottis as the ratchet is braced to allow the assembly to become stable.
3. Figure 19.8 shows the microscope in place for the performance of micro-laryngoscopy. Note the laryngoscopic suspension and the camera and side arm to the microscope which allow for teaching and recording purposes.
4. To remove an area of granulation from a vocal cord the surgeon will grasp the lesion in the cupped forceps and distract it medially and then dissect the lesion out with the use of microscissors.

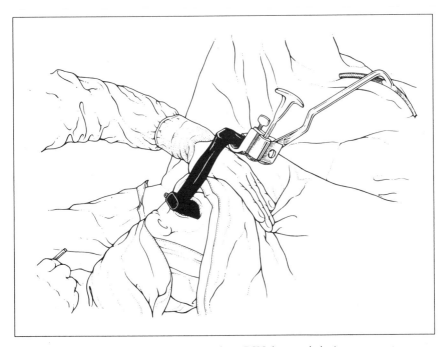

Figure 19.7   Suspension of the laryngoscope (from RSN, by permission)

Laser microlaryngoscopy

The CO_2 laser can be added to the microlaryngoscopic set-up. With the patient and staff, suitably protected against accidental laser strikes, lesions within the larynx can be vaporized.

It is crucial that the surgeon using the laser is aware of the histological diagnosis of the lesion that is being treated. Consequently, in the management of any dysplastic lesion within the larynx a histological biopsy should be performed prior to using the laser.

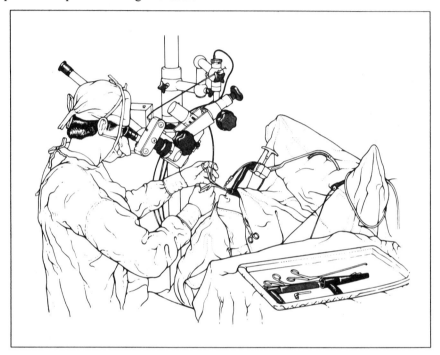

Figure 19.8   The working position for microlaryngoscopy (from RSN, by permission)

Post-operative care

1. Many anaesthetists spray the vocal cords with local anaesthetic agents prior to awakening the patient to ensure that the patient does not go into laryngospasm in the recovery room. This can easily be performed by spraying 4% Xylocaine through the laryngoscope.
2. Potential airway obstruction should be identified during the time of the surgery and a tracheostomy inserted if appropriate.
3. Very occasionally persistent bleeding may require the patient is reassessed under anaesthetic and the bleeding controlled.
4. The specific aftercare will often be determined by the lesion which is being treated within the larynx. Voice rest is appropriate for most endolaryngeal surgery. If the patient is going to talk he or she should talk in a normal voice as whispering may strain the voice further.
5. Appropriate arrangements to review the histology with the patient should always be made.

RIGID BRONCHOSCOPY

Indications

1. To remove foreign bodies or mucous plugs.
2. To evaluate the tracheobronchial tree and to biopsy a suspected tumour.
3. To secure an airway in cases of upper respiratory tract obstruction when intubation is difficult or impossible.

Pre-operative considerations

Recent plain radiographs of the chest should be available. The correct size of bronchoscope should be identified prior to surgery. Figure 19.9 shows the external diameters of bronchoscopes related to their internal dimensions and the age of the patients. Figure 19.2 gives an overview of tracheobronchial anatomy.

Size marked on bronchoscope (MM)	External diameter (MM)	Age range
2.5	4.0	Premature/neonate
3.0	5.0	Neonate–3 months
3.5	5.7	4–12 months
4.0	7.0	12–36 months
5.0	7.8	3–9 years
6.0	8.2	Over 9 years

Figure 19.9 Bronchoscopes used for children, relating the size of instrument to the age of the child (from PO, by permission)

Risks

1. Haemorrhage. A vascular tumour may bleed briskly. If this occurs the head should be tilted downwards and pressure applied with a swab soaked in 1:1000 adrenaline. If this is ineffective a pack, such as a Thompson's blocker or a Fogarty balloon catheter, should be used to compress the site of bleeding. The pack should be left in place for approximately 5 minutes. An aortic aneurysm may rarely be biopsied!
2. Laryngeal oedema as a result of prolonged or rough bronchoscopy.
3. Damage to dentition.
4. Pneumothorax from extensive biopsies.
5. Failure to retrieve foreign bodies. In some circumstances this may require that a thoracotomy is performed to retrieve such a foreign body.
6. On occasion it can be anatomically difficult to insert the bronchoscope. The Negus laryngoscope can be used to identify the larynx and to guide the bronchoscope through the vocal cords. The removal of the lower part of

the laryngoscope allows the surgeon to remove the entire laryngoscope while keeping the bronchoscope in place.

Preparation

This should be discussed with the anaesthetist prior to the procedure. General anaesthesia created with intravenous scoline and pentothal while ventilation is maintained by the oxygen Venturi system attached to the bronchoscope is one method. The patient is supine on the table with the cervical spine flexed and the head extended.

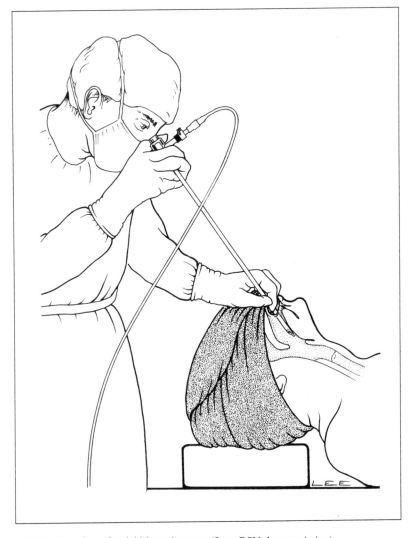

Figure 19.10   Insertion of a rigid bronchoscope (from RSN, by permission)

Method

1. A shield is inserted to protect upper dentition or alternatively a swab is laid over the upper alveolus in those patients without teeth.
2. Figure 19.10 shows the initial insertion of the bronchoscope. It is inserted through the right side of the mouth, lifting and following the tongue to the epiglottis. The tip of the bronchoscope is used to elevate the tip of the epiglottis and gently rotating the bronchoscope allows the glottis to come into view.
3. The bronchoscope is advanced towards the glottis and then rotated through 90° with the tip to the right. Figure 19.11 shows this manoeuvre.

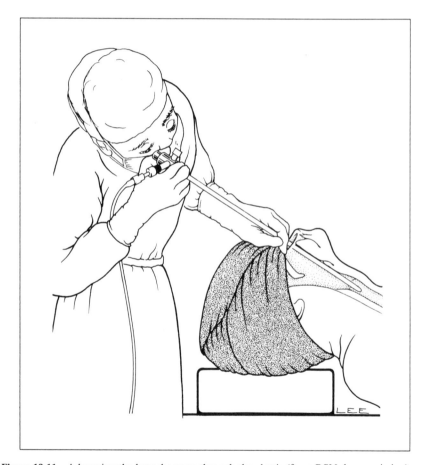

Figure 19.11   Advancing the bronchoscope through the glottis (from RSN, by permission)

4. The view through the bronchoscope is centred on the left vocal cord and the instrument is slowly advanced towards this until the beak passes between the vocal cords. A gentle rotation back through 90° and the bronchoscope has passed the larynx. This is shown in Figure 19.12.

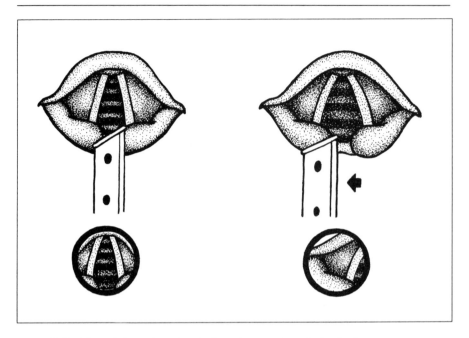

Figure 19.12　The technique of passing the bronchoscope through the glottis

5. Once the surgeon has passed the bronchoscope into the trachea the anaesthetist should fit the Venturi oxygen supply to the side arm of the bronchoscope and the surgeon should fit the glass lens to the proximal end of the bronchoscope. This prevents gas being blown in the face of the surgeon and allows the oxygen to reach the appropriate areas.

6. The bronchoscope is kept in a direct line with the trachea and is advanced slowly, viewing the tracheal walls and the normally sharp outline of the carina.

7. To enter the left main bronchus it is necessary to position the bronchoscope in the right corner of the mouth with the head rotated slightly to the right, bringing the long axis of the instrument and the left main bronchus into alignment. Figure 19.13 demonstrates the view into the left main bronchus.

8. To enter the right main bronchus the instrument and the head are rotated to the left to allow the bronchoscope and right main bronchus to lie in alignment. Figure 19.14 demonstrates the view into the right main bronchus.

9. The use of Hopkin's rod rigid telescope, particularly the 70° version, is very useful for inspecting the entrances of the segmental bronchi. In particular the right upper bronchus requires a lateral viewing telescope for adequate inspection.

10. Any material aspirated through the bronchoscope can be collected for cytology and culture. Endobronchial biopsies can be obtained and for this it is often helpful to use the integral telescope and biopsy forceps.

11. Inert foreign bodies should be withdrawn into the scope. Occasionally large foreign bodies have to be broken down prior to being extracted.

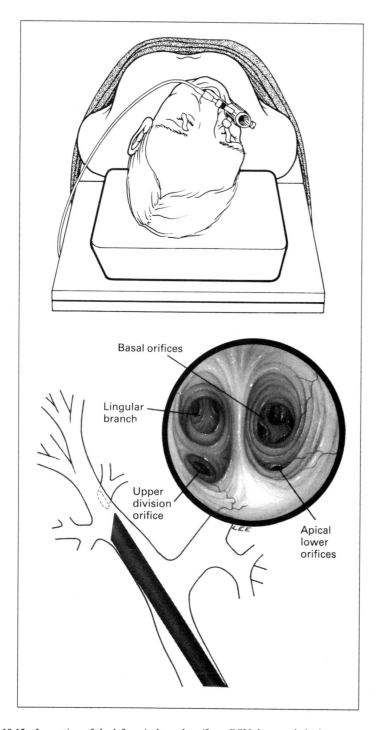

Figure 19.13 Inspection of the left main bronchus (from RSN, by permission)

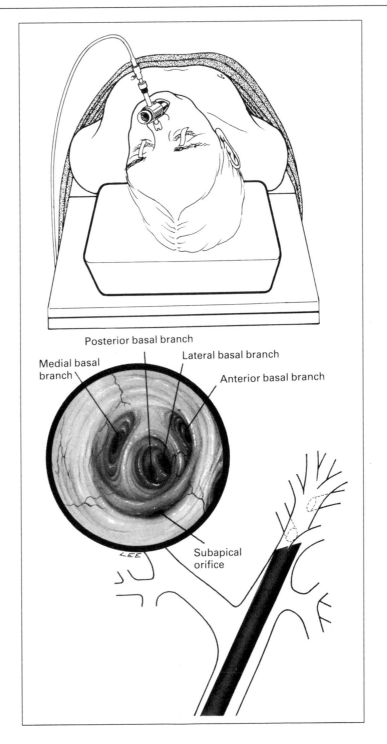

Figure 19.14   Inspection of right main bronchus (from RSN, by permission)

After the removal of an inert foreign body the tracheobronchial tree should be re-examined to ensure that there is no residual debris.
12. Vegetable foreign bodies can be particularly difficult to remove from the tracheobronchial tree as a result of mucosal swelling. This can make extraction of the foreign body difficult. Telescopic forceps are appropriate for removing such foreign bodies.

Post-operative care

1. A surgeon should limit the time of a rigid bronchoscopy to maximally 20 minutes. Manipulation and abrasion of the vocal cords should be avoided.
2. Prolonged bronchoscopy can result in post-operative laryngeal oedema and consequent respiratory obstruction. Spraying the vocal cords with 4% lignocaine at the end of a bronchoscopy can help to prevent post-operative laryngospasm. If laryngeal oedema occurs, then steroids and humidification are necessary.
3. When extensive endobronchial biopsies are performed a post-operative chest X-ray should be arranged to identify any pneumothorax.

RIGID OESOPHAGOSCOPY

Indications

1. Rigid oesophagoscopy is indicated to inspect and obtain biopsies from lesions within the oesophagus. Dysphagia is the cardinal symptom investigated by rigid oesophagoscopy.
2. Foreign bodies lodged in the oesophagus can be removed by rigid oesophagoscopy.
3. Oesophagoscopy is an integral part of panendoscopic investigation of a cervical lymph node considered to contain squamous cell metastatic cancer.
4. Oesophagoscopy may be therapeutic when combined with dilatation by bougies for strictures or for placement of indwelling tubes.
5. A preliminary oesophagoscopy to insert acroflavine gauze is performed in the treatment of pharyngeal pouch.

Specimen

This should be obtained with punch forceps. When the lesion is a post-cricoid carcinoma, or if Patterson/Brown–Kelly (Plummer/Vinson) syndrome is suspected a full blood count and film are required.

Pre-operative considerations

1. It is, usually, wise to have a barium swallow performed prior to endoscopy

for chronic dysphagia. This allows an unexpected pharyngeal pouch to be identified or a prominent aortic knuckle shown. The barium swallow may also direct the surgeon to examine a particular area of the oesophagus.

2. If the problem is an ingested foreign body then plain soft tissue radiographs of the neck plus plain radiographs both in the P.A. and lateral view are required to identify the site of the foreign body.

3. Typically a foreign body will arrest at the anatomical and physiological narrowings within the oesophagus. Specifically these are:
   - The cricopharyngeus muscle (15 cm from the incisor teeth).
   - The aortic arch (22.5 cm from the incisor teeth).
   - The left main bronchus (27.5 cm from the incisor teeth).
   - The diaphragm (40 cm from the incisor teeth). (N.B. distances are approximate for an average adult male).

4. When there is doubt as to the mobility of the patient's cervical spine, a lateral soft tissue will be helpful. Prominent cervical osteophytes can cause considerable difficulty in the insertion of the oesophagoscope.

5. In some circumstances, such as kyphoscoliosis or spinal rigidity as a result of ankylosing spondylitis, rigid oesophagoscopy may not be possible.

6. A pre-operative note should be made of the state of the patient's dentition. There is always a risk of damaging or dislodging teeth during the performance of an oesophagoscopy and the patient should be warned of this.

Risks

1. Damage to the lips and teeth.
2. Haematoma of the posterior pharyngeal wall.
3. Perforation of the oesophagus or pharynx.
4. Failure to obtain an appropriate biopsy.

Preparation

1. General per-oral endotracheal anaesthesia is the most common anaesthetic for rigid oesophagoscopy. It is possible to perform rigid oesophagoscopy under local anaesthetic, but this is rarely performed.

2. The patient is supine on the table with a pillow under the shoulders, giving some support to the head, which is extended at the atlanto-occipital joint. This is the 'sniffing of the morning air' position. Alternatively, a special table with head supports can be used.

Method

1. The teeth are protected with a shield, or in an edentulous patient a gauze swab is put over the upper alveolus.

2. The oesophagoscope is held in the surgeon's right hand and introduced through the right side of the mouth while the surgeon with his or her left hand retracts the lips and protects the teeth. It is often necessary to aspirate excessive saliva from the back of the pharynx.

3. The surgeon identifies the endotracheal tube as it passes the epiglottis and then follows down the right hand side of the endotracheal tube beyond the epiglottis. The oesophagoscope passes down towards the right pyriform fossa and then slips behind the endotracheal tube to identify the crico-pharyngeal sphincter.

4. The tip of the oesophagoscope is advanced into the centre of cricopharyn-geus and then as gentle pressure is applied the oesophagus opens in front of the examiner.

5. It can on occasion be difficult to pass an oesophagoscope through crico-pharyngeus. The surgeon should check for three points:
   - Has the anaesthetist given the patient sufficient muscle relaxant.
   - The surgeon should consider whether there are large osteophytes causing an obstructive difficulty. If this is the case then manipulation of the scope from the pyriform fossa into the upper oesophagus is required.
   - The cuff of the endotracheal tube may be causing compression of the upper oesophagus.

6. Once the scope is into the oesophagus then alteration of the position of the head of the patient is required to keep the lumen of the oesophagus in full view as the scope is progressively passed downwards to the stomach.

7. To remove a sharp foreign body from the oesophagus it is necessary to grasp the object with the forceps and then withdraw the foreign body into the lumen of the oesophagoscope prior to withdrawing both the foreign body and the oesophagoscope together. It is imperative that a sharp object does not project laterally beyond the edge of the oesophagoscope as this may potentially damage the entire lining of the oesophagus. Soft foreign bodies can be removed piecemeal. Occasionally certain foreign bodies require shears to divide them (dentures) before removal. Rarely special forceps are required to close safety pins before these are removed.

8. Biopsies should be taken with punch forceps. Twisting and pulling actions which may result in perforation of the oesophagus should be avoided.

9. In the management of benign osesophageal strictures bouginage is helpful. Gradual dilatation by using progressively larger gum elastic oesophageal bougies is appropriate. The dilatation should be by gentle pressure rather than undue force.

Post-operative care

1. Perforation is the most serious complication of oesophagoscopy. The patient should be monitored regularly for the development of surgical emphysema within the neck, severe pain in the neck, breathlessness, and intra-abdominal pain. Where there is any doubt a chest X-ray should be performed.

   If a perforation occurs then intravenous antibiotics, nil by mouth, and surgical exploration (depending on the precise site) may be required.

2. It is important to remember that the distal end of the oesophagus is intra-abdominal. Perforation of the lower end may result in a clinical picture of an acute abdominal emergency.

3. After 6 hours the patient should be commenced on sterile fluids. Normal fluids and diet can usually be commenced the following day.
4. The long-term aftercare of an oesophagoscopy depends on the pathology found and treated.

DOHLMANN'S PROCEDURE (DIATHERMY TREATMENT OF A PHARYNGEAL POUCH)

Indications

In particularly frail individuals, as an alternative to an external approach, in the treatment of pharyngeal pouch, diathermy and division of the party wall between the pouch and the oesophagus, as described originally by Dohlmann, is a useful operation.

Pre-operative considerations

1. The tissue divided includes the circular fibres of the cricopharyngeus muscle.
2. It is worth reading the chapter on external approaches to pharyngeal pouch as many of the pre-operative considerations are the same.
3. The patient should be in a good state of nutrition and any overspill chest infection as a result of the pouch should be treated prior to surgery. In cases of a large pouch the pouch should be washed out before surgery.
4. It is crucial to have the instruments which were specifically designed by Dohlmann for this operation. These consist of:
   - A special endoscope split distally to provide an anterior lip which passes into the oesophagus and a posterior lip which passes into the pouch.
   - Insulated diathermy forceps.
   - Diathermy knife.
   - The protector to prevent damage from the diathermy knife.
5. The vocal cord movements should be examined and recorded pre-operatively.
6. A broad spectrum antibiotic cover, such as Augmentin, should be given with the induction of the anaesthetic.

Risks

1. Perforation. This can result in local surgical emphysema and can also result in both local and mediastinal infection. This should be aggressively treated with antibiotics.
2. Vocal cord paralysis has been reported from this operation.
3. Excessive diathermy to the upper oesophagus can result in stenosis, which requires treatment by dilatation.
4. Carcinoma can occur in a pouch which has not been removed. It is, of course, crucial to inspect the pouch fully prior to diathermy treatment.

5. One should always consider the state of a patient's dentition before rigid endoscopy and warn of potential damage.

Preparation

A general anaesthetic is provided through a cuffed oral endotracheal tube with the anaesthetist using non-explosive anaesthetic agents. The patient lies supine with the neck flexed and the head extended.

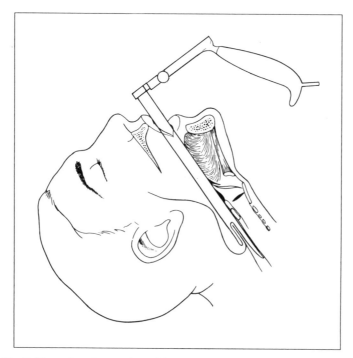

Figure 19.15 Dohlmann's endoscope in position (from RSN, by permission)

Method

1. Dohlmann's endoscope is passed so that its anterior lip passes into the oesophagus and its posterior lip passes into the pouch. Figure 19.15 demonstrates this position.
2. The tissue between the pouch and the oesophagus presents as a bar on inspection through the endoscope. This ridge is grasped with a specially insulated diathermy forceps and a coagulating current is applied for 1 to 2 minutes, or until the tissue turns white, depending on the thickness of the tissue involved. Three forcep widths of tissue are coagulated.

3. The surgeon then passes the insulated protector into the pharyngeal pouch. The coagulated area can now be divided with the diathermy knife cutting backwards onto the protector within the pouch. Adequate division of the party wall between the oesophagus and the pouch concludes the procedure.
4. A nasogastric tube is passed down the oesophagus at the end of operation.

Post-operative care

1. The patient is fed through the nasogastric tube for 5 days and then commenced on diet. It is preferable to start with fluids and work up to a normal diet.
2. The antibiotic cover is maintained until the patient is swallowing satisfactorily, usually at 5 days.

The procedure can be easily repeated. It is therefore better to err on the side of caution in performing this diathermy myotomy.

Chapter 20

Neck surgery

BASIC PRINCIPLES

It is very important to be aware of the pathology of a neck lesion on which one is going to operate. To achieve this one should use all reasonable diagnostic means prior to recourse to surgery. For lateral neck masses preliminary fine needle aspiration biopsy, ultrasound and, on occasion, CT scan of the neck can be useful. If there is suspicion that the lateral neck mass may be a squamous cell carcinoma then a chest X-ray plus a panendoscopy and examination of the post-nasal space are mandatory prior to removal of the mass. When the diagnostic suspicion is for a lymphoma then examination of the other lymph node-bearing sites in the body plus palpation for enlarged liver and the spleen are essential.

For mid-line neck masses which encroach on the thyroid gland a thyroid isotope scan, diagnostic ultrasound scan, thyroid antibodies and a CT scan of the neck can all be useful.

In general, the success of neck surgery will largely be determined by the pathological diagnosis. Poor surgical technique, however, can always worsen the situation for the patient.

Incision planning

If one is planning to excise a lump as a diagnostic procedure then in planning the incision one should consider that either yourself or another surgeon may have to return at a later date to perform a far wider excision. A specific example of this would be a radical neck dissection to treat squamous cell carcinoma of the lymph nodes of the neck. The 'lumpectomy' incision, therefore, should be designed in such a way that it can be encompassed in a radical neck incision.

Cosmesis is always an important part of neck incisions. In general, transverse skin crease incisions have a cosmetically superior appearance. It is important, however, that the relatively small gain of post-operative cosmetic appearance is not sacrificed at the expense of inadequate surgical exposure and consequently an inadequately performed operation. A specific example of this would be a transverse incision versus an incision along the anterior sternomastoid border in the external approach to a pharyngeal pouch. The vertical incision gives far better exposure for the surgeon in training. It is also important that many of these patients are elderly and as a result the laxity and wrinkles within the skin will have less obvious scars.

Vertical incisions in the lateral part of the neck are prone to form webs as they heal. It is for this reason that the lower vertical limb of a radical neck dissection should either be in the shape of an 's' or have a hitch in it.

Simple 'lumpectomy' in the neck should be considered a misnomer. The lymph nodes of the neck almost always lie in close proximity to the jugular vein and therefore one should never approach a lump biopsy of the neck lightly.

Surgical technique

Bad surgical technique can always worsen the lot for a patient. One should avoid mishandling skin and flaps with fingers or applying toothed forceps to skin edges. The division of the skin should be at right-angles. The surgeon should divide directly and straight through platysma. In general, neck flaps for exposure are raised in the subplatysmal plane. There are schools of support for elevating neck flaps by scalpel dissection and by scissor dissection. In the irradiated patient knife dissection is easier. Meticulous control of haemorrhage is important. A wound should always be thoroughly checked at the end of an operation to ensure that no bleeding spots are present.

It is always worthwhile checking that the anaesthetist has returned the blood pressure completely to normal if hypotensive techniques have been used during head and neck surgery. If this is not done than a haematoma can often form rapidly after the operation as the blood pressure returns to normal.

There is some evidence that blood transfusion during a resection for head and neck cancer may worsen the prognosis of the patient. Currently this evidence is debated because the need for blood may indicate:

1. Poor surgical technique.
2. Extensive disease.
3. Some other, as yet unidentifiable, factor.

Drainage

A suction drain should be inserted whenever there is a dead space in the neck at the end of the operation. The drain should be removed when there is a minimum of drainage. This means when there is less than 10 ml in the preceding 24 hours. Suction drains should always be brought out through a separate stab incision and it is often wise to both suture the drain in position and to apply sticky tape to ensure that the drains are not pulled out accidentally. A wound has to be adequately sealed for a suction drain to work effectively. The most important layer for an airtight seal of the wound is the platysmal layer. This layer should be closed either with an interrupted or continuous absorbable suture such as a 3-0 chronic catgut.

When siting drains one should take care not to allow the fenestra (through which the liquid is aspirated) of the drain to lie over any major vessels. One may have to put a small stitch of catgut within the wound to hold the drain in the correct position.

Wound haemostasis

A surgeon may use either bipolar or unipolar diathermy to secure haemostasis within the neck. One should try to limit the use of non-absorbable sutures deep within the wound as these may result in small abscesses. When an artery has been ligated within the neck and there is any doubt as to the security of the ligature it is often wisest to suture ligate that particular vessel.

Prophylactic antibiotics

If the pharynx, larynx or oesophagus are going to be opened surgically then the patient should have a prophylactic antibiotic. Amoxycillin with clavulanic acid effectively covers most of the potentially infecting organisms and can be given as an intravenous dose at the time of induction of the anaesthetic. There is argument as to the time period of the antibiotic cover. This will depend on the precise nature of the surgery and the individual wishes of the surgeon.

Nasogastric tubes

Nasogastric tubes are routinely inserted following laryngectomy, pharyngectomy, pharyngeal pouch excision and Dohlmann's procedure. There are a number of ways to secure a nasogastric tube in position, which means that there is no universally satisfactory method. The tube may be sutured to the nasal columella, taped or plastered to the forehead and nose, or suspended via a rubber catheter which is inserted through one nostril and brought out through the other. The most important feature, however, is to ensure that the nasogastric tube does not come out accidentally. The reinsertion of a nasogastric tube shortly after a total laryngectomy can cause considerable damage to the pharyngeal suture layer.

Skin closure

Careful skin handling is essential. Closure can be with interrupted non-absorbable sutures, a subcuticular repair or with the use of staples or clips. When non-absorbable sutures or staples are used, they should be removed before they can cause cross-hatch marks.

After about 2 weeks cold cream or wheatgerm oil should be smoothed along the incision and any crusts removed from the wound. This helps to soften the incision. For the first 6 months to 1 year wounds are prone to an angry erythematous reaction to strong sunlight. The patient should, therefore, wear a strong sun factor cream to avoid this happening. Factor 10 to 14 is adequate.

TRACHEOSTOMY

Indications

There are two principal types of indication for tracheostomy. The first is upper airway obstruction and the second is to provide ventilatory support. These indications can be sub-divided into:

A. Upper airway obstruction:
    1. Congenital:
        - Subglottic stenosis.
        - Sleep apnoea syndrome.
        - Treacher-Collins.
        - Laryngeal web.
    2. Accidental trauma
        - Maxillary and mandibular fractures.
        - Laryngeal injuries.
        - Foreign bodies in the airway.
        - Prolonged or traumatic endotracheal intubation.
    3. Neoplasia
        - Laryngeal and pharyngeal tumours.
        - Malignant thyroid tumours.
    4. Infective problems
        - Acute epiglottis.
        - Acute laryngitis.
        - Deep neck space infections.
    5. Inflammation
        - Angioneurotic oedema.
        - Oedema as a result of inhalation of smoke, fumes or corrosive agents.
    6. Neurological problems
        - Pharyngeal or laryngeal paralysis as a result of motor neurone disease.
        - Bilateral recurrent laryngeal nerve paralysis (thyroid surgery).
        - Myasthenia gravis.
    7. Surgery on the upper airway, particularly major resections within the oral cavity and pharynx.

B. To provide ventilatory support:
    1. Head injuries.
    2. Coma from narcotic or drug overdose.
    3. As respiratory support following thoracic procedures.
    4. Flail chest.
    5. To allow access to the lower airways to facilitate removal of excess secretions.
    6. Severe pneumonia.
    7. Acute or chronic bronchitis.
    8. Tetanus.

Specimen

If one is performing the procedure to relieve obstruction due to laryngeal or pharyngeal tumours and a section is to be cut from the trachea then the specimen should be sent to pathology to ensure that there is no extension of the tumour to the site of the tracheostomy.

Pre-operative considerations

A patient should be warned that he or she may not be able to produce voice immediately following the operation.

Risks

1. *Haemorrhage*

This can occur immediately following the operation and is typically from cutaneous vessels. Other sources of bleeding include the anterior jugular veins, the thyroid isthmus and from the tracheal wall. If secondary bleeding occurs (more than 5 days after the initial operation) then a cuffed tube should be inserted as an emergency measure and the wound reopened to control the haemorrhage. An ill-fitting tracheostomy tube can erode through the anterior wall of the trachea and damage a large vessel.

2. *Apnoea*

This may occur if a patient has been surviving on carbon dioxide respiratory drive (hypoxic drive). The opening of the trachea may result in an abrupt decrease in the carbon dioxide content in the blood and as a result stimulus for breathing may disappear. An administration of 5% carbon dioxide and oxygen may be necessary for a few hours after the opening of the trachea.

3. *Subcutaneous emphysema and pneumothorax*

These complications are more common in children. Avoiding the tight closure round the tracheostomy tube is important to prevent the emphysema and unnecessary dissection in the tissue planes should avoid the creation of a pneumothorax. If the pleura is accidentally damaged then it should be closed at the time of operation.

4. *Obstruction of the tube*

Adequate humidification is important to prevent tenacious secretions obstructing the tube. Regular suction helps prevent the complication of tube obstruction. When there is an inner tube this can be removed and changed in cases of obstruction. If a tube cannot be adequately cleaned then it has to be replaced by a fresh one.

5.   Tube dislodgement

Suture of the flanges of the tube to the skin or the correct use of tracheostomy tapes should avoid dislodgement of the tube.

6.   Pulmonary infection

Excessive bronchial secretions usually occur as a result of the irritation of the tracheostomy tube and the exposure of the trachea to non-humidified air.

7.   Decannulation difficulty

This most typically occurs with children and their dependence on the tracheostomy may be decreased by gradually reducing the size of the tracheostomy tube and partly occluding the tube.

8.   Tracheal stenosis

Damage to the first ring of the trachea predisposes to subglottic stenosis.

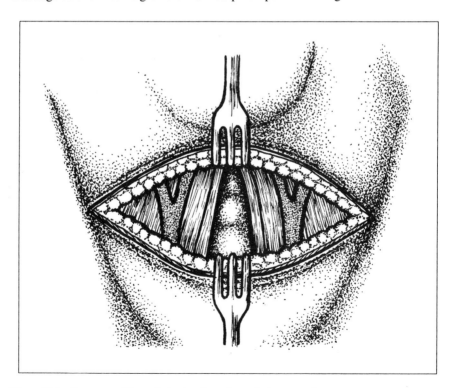

Figure 20.1   Exposure of the anterior jugular veins and strap muscles

Preparation

An elective procedure is ideally performed under a general peroral endotracheal anaesthesia. If there is such upper airway obstruction that an endotracheal tube cannot be passed then local anaesthesia with 1% lignocaine and 1:200 000 adrenaline is used. Immediately prior to opening the trachea 0.5 ml of 4% lignocaine should be injected into the tracheal lumen.

In the elective procedure a sandbag is placed under the patient's shoulder to give extension to the neck and prominence to the trachea and larynx. When a patient has severe dyspnoea and the procedure is performed under a local anaesthetic then a compromise position of extension may be required.

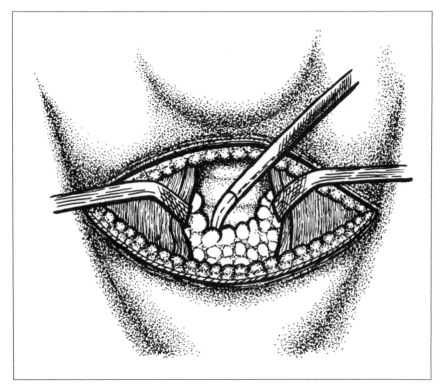

Figure 20.2   Development of plane of dissection between the thyroid isthmus and trachea using an artery clip

Method

1. A small transverse incision approximately midway between the cricoid cartilage and the suprasternal notch (approximately 2 cm below the lower border of the cricoid cartilage) is deepened through skin, subcutaneous fat and deep cervical fascia. Figure 20.1 demonstrates the initial exposure. The mid-line raphe between the right and left strap muscles is divided to reveal the thyroid gland and upper part of the trachea.
2. In most patients the thyroid isthmus has to be divided to give good access to the anterior wall of the trachea. A small incision is created in the midline at the lower border of the cricoid cartilage through the pre-tracheal fascia. This allows a small clip to be inserted and directed inferiorly behind

the thyroid isthmus and the trachea. This plane can then be opened by blunt dissection. Figure 20.2 shows the initial insinuation of the artery clip.

3. A large artery clip is placed on either side of the thyroid isthmus, which is then divided with a knife. The cut surfaces of the thyroid are oversewn (Figure 20.3).

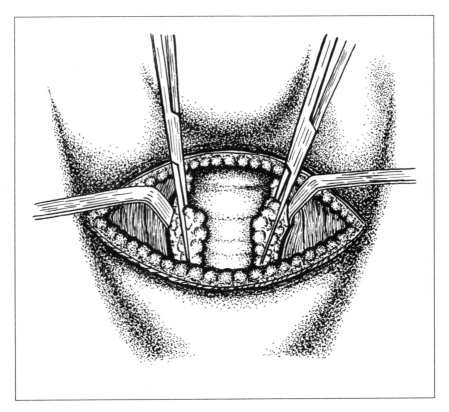

Figure 20.3   The cut surfaces of the thyroid are oversewn

4. Prior to opening the trachea haemostasis should be complete. A sucker should be to hand to aspirate from the trachea and the appropriate tracheostomy tube chosen for insertion. A cricoid hook inserted under the cricoid cartilage can be of use in elevating the trachea to the surface of the wound.

5. A vertical incision or a circle incision can be made into the anterior wall of the trachea, usually at the level of the second and third tracheal rings. The first ring should not be damaged. Figure 20.4 demonstrates these points. Note the access given by division of the thyroid isthmus.

6. Following insertion, the cuff of the tube is inflated and anaesthesia continues through the cuffed tracheostomy tube. The wound is closed, avoiding excessive tension on the sutures. A tight closure of this wound predisposes to surgical emphysema.

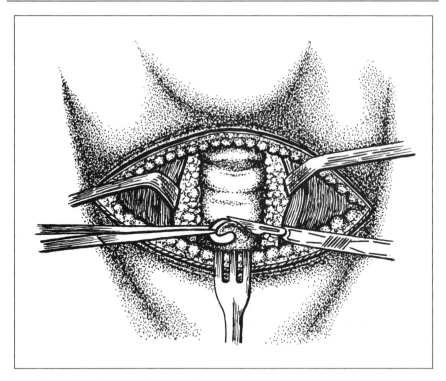

Figure 20.4 A window of cartilage is excised from the anterior wall of the trachea

7. To secure the tracheostomy tube the flanges may be sutured to the skin with a stout non-absorbable suture. Alternatively, the tapes of the tracheostomy may be sufficient for security. To tie the tapes it is important that the patient's head is well flexed when the knots are tied, otherwise the ties may become slack when the patient sits up in bed, resulting in dislodgement of the tube. A preformed dressing is usually inserted under and around the tracheostomy tube.
8. In some circumstances, particularly in children, where there is danger of losing the tracheostomy tube, it is worthwhile inserting non-absorbable nylon sutures in the trachea on either side of the opening to facilitate emergency tube reinsertion.

Modifications of the technique for young children

1. In infants the larynx is relatively higher in the neck than in the adult. It is not uncommon to find the innominate vein rising into the jugular notch, particularly with the effort of obstructed breathing. Care should be taken to avoid damaging it.
2. In babies the domes of the pleura are paratracheal in the neck. The pleura can easily be damaged, with the risk of pneumothorax.
3. The trachea should always be opened with a vertical slit. Resection of cartilage is associated with a very high incidence of subsequent tracheal stenosis.

Modifications of the technique in an emergency

Clearly if the patient is severely cyanosed, or has in fact totally stopped breathing, speed is of the essence. At all costs the airway must be opened. The niceties of technique are dropped. In the situation where seconds count, do not waste time with:

1. Scrubbing up.
2. Local anaesthesia.
3. Controlling haemorrhage – use the sucker.
4. Clipping and dividing the thyroid isthmus – just cut straight through it.
5. Identifying laryngeal landmarks – just slit open the airway in the midline with a vertical incision.

It is better to save the patient's life than to lose it worrying about complications such as delayed tracheal stenosis.

Post-operative care

1. It is crucial that the tracheostomy tube must not become dislodged or obstructed. The tension of the securing tapes must be regularly checked, or alternatively the tube must be sutured to the skin.
2. A soft tissue radiograph of the neck will confirm the correct position of the tube.
3. The cuff of the tube should be released after approximately 24 hours, unless the patient is being ventilated.
4. Adequate humidification should be supplied. Secretions should be removed from the trachea and bronchi with a soft sterile catheter.
5. The patient will not be able to speak when the cuff of the tube is inflated and may also, in this circumstance, have some difficulty in swallowing.
6. The first tube change should take place after about 4–5 days, when a track is well formed. The first change should be performed by the surgeon who created the tracheostomy with the patient in the same position as he or she was to create the tracheostomy. Good illumination and suction are necessary.
7. Once the tube is changed a tube with a speaking valve may be inserted to allow the return of normal voice.

EXCISION OF A THYROGLOSSAL DUCT CYST

Indications

A thyroglossal duct cyst occurs along the line of migration of the embryonic thyroid and can lie anywhere between the foramen caecum and the thyroid isthmus. This cyst should be excised either for cosmetic reasons or following infection of the cyst.

Specimen

The cyst, the body of the hyoid and the persistent thyroglossal duct upwards to the foramen caecum.

Pre-operative considerations

Incision and drainage of an infected thyroglossal cyst should be avoided, as subsequent surgery is more difficult. In this circumstance an ellipse of skin through which the previous drainage has been performed is excised at the time of operation.

Many surgeons arrange a thyroid isotope scan to determine the disposition of all thyroid tissue prior to surgery.

Risks

1. The commonest problem is that part of the cyst or the thyroglossal duct is left behind leading to a recurrence. Surgery for a recurrence is inevitably difficult. As a consequence the cyst plus the body of the hyoid and the thyroglossal duct from the foramen caecum should always be removed at the primary operation.
2. Wound haematoma.

Preparation

General anaesthesia delivered through a nasotracheal tube. The patient is supine on the table, with the neck extended by a small pillow under the shoulders and the head stabilized on a head ring.

Method

1. A collar incision in a skin crease centred over the upper part of the cyst is usually adequate. This would typically be at the level of the thyroid prominence and is shown in Figure 20.5. The incision is deepened through platysma and subplatysmal flaps elevated.
2. The cyst is dissected free from the strap muscles and the persistent thyroglossal duct followed towards the hyoid bone. The muscular attachments to the central segment of the hyoid bone are detached and the body of the hyoid is divided with bone cutters and a segment of approximately 1–2 cm wide removed.
3. With a finger in the mouth and pressure on the foramen caecum, a conical shape of muscle is excised from the base of the tongue between the hyoid bone and the foramen caecum in order to remove the most superior part of a persistent thyroglossal duct. Figure 20.6 demonstrates the cyst, the body of the hyoid and the thyroglossal duct being removed from the base of the tongue.

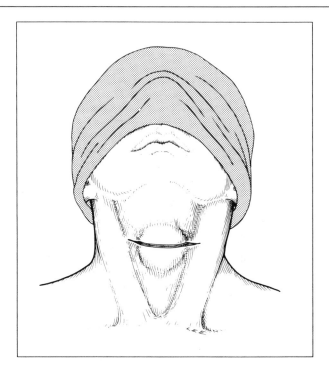

Figure 20.5 Site of incision for exploration of a thyroglossal cyst (from RSN, by permission)

4. The defect in the base of the tongue is closed by approximating the muscle. A suction drain is inserted and the wound is closed in two layers with absorbable sutures to close platysma and then non-absorbable sutures or clips to the skin.

Post-operative care

The drain is removed when there is minimal drainage.

THYROIDECTOMY

Indications

1. Extensive papillary carcinoma, follicular carcinoma and medullary carcinoma of the thyroid are often best treated by total thyroidectomy.
2. A cold nodule of the thyroid in which the histological diagnosis is uncertain is often preferably treated by a thyroid lobectomy.
3. Grave's disease or primary thyrotoxicosis can be treated by a subtotal thyroidectomy.

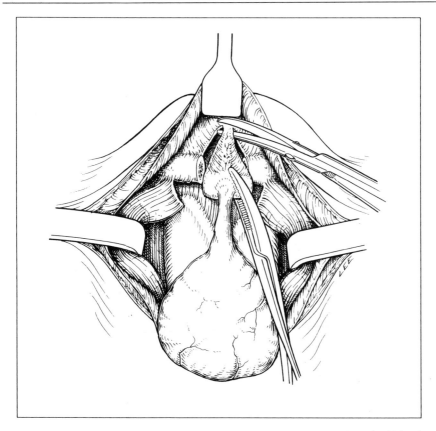

Figure 20.6 Exposure of the cyst and thyroglossal duct. Note the body of the hyoid has been divided (from RSN, by permission)

4. A thyroid lobectomy or total thyroidectomy may be done in the course of a radical operation to remove squamous cell carcinoma within the larynx, pharynx or upper oesophagus.
5. A multinodular goitre may be removed for cosmetic reasons.

Specimen

Thyroid gland.

Pre-operative considerations

The appropriate investigations of a thyroid mass should be available prior to surgery. This would normally include a thyroid isotope scan, ultrasound or on occasion a CT scan of the neck. Thyroid function tests and a baseline serum calcium should be performed. In those patients undergoing thyroidectomy to treat thyrotoxicosis, close liaison with the endocrinologist is essential. The patient is usually prepared for surgery with a combination of antithyroid drugs and beta blockers.

The vocal cords should be inspected prior to thyroidectomy to ensure that both recurrent nerves are functioning normally. Plain radiographs of the thoracic inlet are often useful to identify any compression of the trachea by the thyroid gland.

In a total thyroidectomy a bilateral lobectomy is performed, although one must ensure that the thyroid isthmus is removed. In a subtotal thyroidectomy for thyroitoxicosis a close search is made to identify the parathyroid glands. These are typically related to the thyroid arterial pedicles. One parathyroid gland may be found close to where the inferior thyroid artery enters the thyroid and another close to where the superior thyroid artery enters the gland. Once identified, the parathyroids are preserved. A bloodless field facilitates identification of the parathyroid glands. In the subtotal thyroidectomy a rim of thyroid tissue is left at the isthmus. This usually is between 5 and 10 g in volume.

Risks

1. Haematoma (this can precipitate airway obstruction).
2. Hypocalcaemia.
3. Hypothyroidism.
4. Unsightly scar.
5. Superior laryngeal nerve palsy.
6. Unilateral recurrent nerve palsy. This is often not identified for a number of months after surgery.
7. Bilateral recurrent nerve palsy. Occasionally this is not noted following surgery until the patient suddenly develops airway obstruction.

Preparation

The patient receives general anaesthesia through an oral or nasal endotracheal tube. The patient is supine on the table with a sandbag under the shoulder to extend the neck and a head ring placed under the head for security.

Method

1. A thyroid lobectomy will be described.
2. A collar incision centred over the thyroid is marked out. The incision is deepened through platysma and then superior and inferior subplatysmal flaps are elevated. The upper flap is raised to the level of the thyroid cartilage and the lower flap to the level of the upper border of the sternum. The flaps are retracted by using a Joll's thyroid retractor.
3. The strap muscles are divided vertically in the midline of the neck and they are then retracted laterally with dissection proceeding in the plane between the gland and the muscles. Alternatively, these muscles are divided low in the neck and reflected laterally from the thyroid lobe.

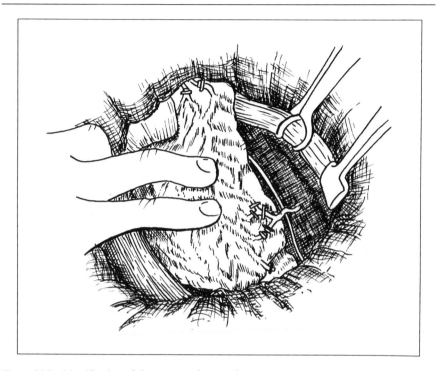

Figure 20.7 Identification of the recurrent laryngeal nerve

4. The next step is to identify and preserve the recurrent laryngeal nerve. The recurrent laryngeal nerve lies in the groove between the trachea and the oesophagus. Careful dissection posteriorly next to the wall of the trachea and inferior to the thyroid isthmus should allow identification of the recurrent nerve. The initial identification of the nerve is shown in Figure 20.7. Once the nerve is identified it should be traced upwards, with the use of artery clip dissection, lifting the gland free as shown in Figure 20.8. Diathermy should be avoided close to the nerve.

5. As the elevation of the gland from the nerve progresses superiorly it will be arrested by the middle thyroid vein, which has to be divided and ligated. This is followed by the inferior thyroid artery. The recurrent nerve has a variable course relative to the inferior thyroid artery and it may run medial, lateral or between the branches of the inferior thyroid artery. A parathyroid gland is often identified at this point. The inferior thyroid artery should be ligated and divided proximally. The proximal end of the artery should be transfixed and ligated. The recurrent nerve should be followed up until it disappears into the larynx.

6. The upper pole of the thyroid is now mobilized with the upper vascular pedicle both ligated and transfixed. Care should be taken, however, as loss of the superior thyroid artery at the upper pole of the thyroid gland can be a serious problem. Damage to the superior laryngeal nerve can occur during division of the upper pole of the thyroid gland. Dissection close to the upper pole of the gland may avoid this problem.

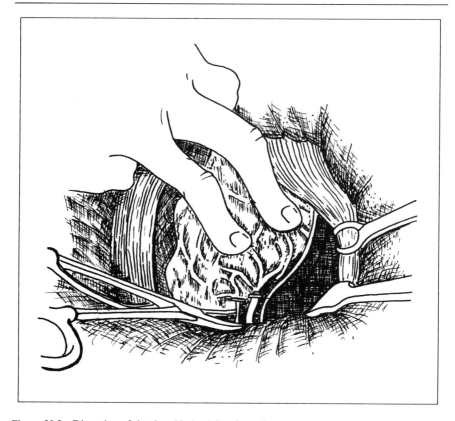

Figure 20.8   Dissection of the thyroid gland free from the nerve

7.   The thyroid isthmus may have to be oversewn to secure haemostasis. A suction drain should always be inserted. In a total thyroidectomy or subtotal thyroidectomy two drains should be inserted with one on either side. If the strap muscles have been divided, attempts may be made to reconstitute them. The wound is closed in two layers with absorbable sutures to platysma and non-absorbable sutures or clips to skin.

Post-operative care

The drains should be removed when there is a minimum of drainage, usually less than 10 ml of blood in the preceding 24 hours. This usually occurs after 48 hours. The serum calcium should be monitored post-operatively. If the patient develops signs of hypocalcaemia then treatment is with infusion of 10% calcium gluconate. Transient hypocalcaemia is not an uncommon post-operative occurrence, even when the parathyroids have been preserved. It is assumed that this is the result of a transient ischaemia to the glands and it will recover.

When there has been complete removal of the thyroid gland and parathyroid glands then the help of an endocrinologist is useful. The patient will require long-term thyroid replacement in addition to calcium supplements.

LIGATURE OF THE EXTERNAL CAROTID ARTERY

Indications

When other methods fail to control bleeding from the mouth, the tongue, the tonsils, the lower two-thirds of the nasal cavity and associated paranasal sinuses, the pharynx and the larynx. This form of severe haemorrhage can result from:

1. Radionecrosis following treatment of malignant disease.
2. Erosion of a major vessel by malignant disease.
3. A surgical procedure.
4. Trauma to the face or neck.
5. Ulcerative non-malignant disease of the head and neck.
6. Spontaneous epistaxis.

Ideally it is preferable to ligate the particular branch of the external carotid artery which results in the haemorrhage, such as the maxillary artery in the pterygopalatine fossa for epistaxis. This, however, is sometimes neither technically possible nor is the precise anatomy of the bleeding known that it is possible to ligate the individual vessel.

Pre-operative considerations

As most of the indications for ligature of the external carotid involve either concurrent or potential severe haemorrhage, cross-matched blood should be available. Following the ligature of the external carotid artery, cross-circulation from the opposite external carotid artery and from the internal carotid artery by communicating branches prevent necrosis of any structures on one side of the head and neck. It is worth considering other possible sources of blood supply to the bleeding site prior to ligature of the external carotid artery as these accessory vessels may require also to be ligated. For example, the anterior ethmoidal artery (from the internal carotid) supplying blood to the nose and the inferior thyroid artery (from the thyrocervical trunk) supplying blood to the larynx.

Risks

1. Damage to the hypoglossal and vagus nerve.
2. Wound haematoma.
3. Failure to control the bleeding due to supply from another source.
4. Injury to structures in the carotid sheath.

Preparation

General anaesthesia delivered through a peroral endotracheal tube with protective packs placed, usually, in the bleeding site. The patient is supine on the table, which is tilted foot-down, and a sandbag placed under the shoulders with the head partly rotated to the opposite side from the surgical procedure.

Method

1. A curved incision in a skin fold of the neck is centred over the bifurcation of the common carotid artery at the upper border of the thyroid cartilage. Alternatively, an incision is made along the anterior border of the sterno-mastoid muscle centred over the upper border of the thyroid cartilage (the landmark for the bifurcation of the common carotid artery).
2. The incision is deepened through the platysma to the deep cervical fascia. At the upper part of either incision one should take care to preserve the greater auricular nerve as it crosses the sternomastoid muscle from inferior to superior. The deep cervical fascia is divided along the anterior border of the sternomastoid muscle and blunt dissection used to expose the carotid artery. The facial vein may require division and ligation. Figure 20.9 demonstrates the relevant anatomy of the carotid artery bifurcation.
3. Opening the carotid sheath demonstrates the common carotid artery, the jugular vein and the vagus nerve which lies posteriorly. The bifurcation of the common carotid artery usually lies at the level of the upper border of the thyroid cartilage. The posterior belly of digastric and the stylohyoid muscle which cross laterally to the internal and external carotid arteries should be identified and retracted superiorly to expose the carotid bulb. This should reveal the hypoglossal nerve as it crosses lateral to both arteries.
4. It is important to identify the external carotid artery by demonstrating two of its branches. It is not unknown for the internal carotid artery, as an anomaly, to have one branch.
5. The external carotid artery is ligated in continuity.
6. The wound is closed in two layers and a small suction drain inserted.

Post-operative care

The drain is removed when there is minimal drainage.

EXCISION OF A BRANCHIAL CYST

Indications

A branchial cyst is a lateral neck cyst which should be excised either for cosmetic reasons or for reasons of recurrent infection and swelling.

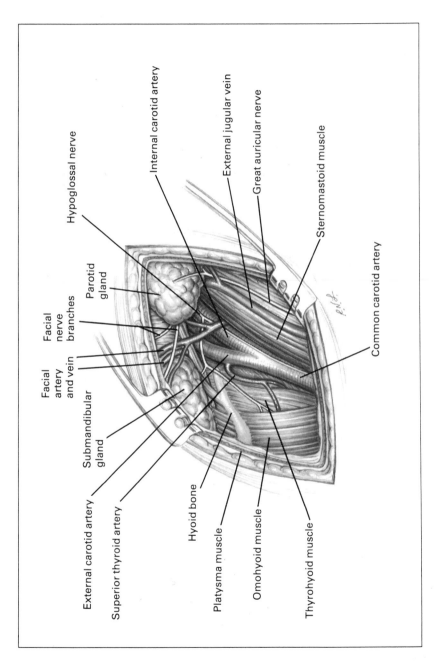

Figure 20.9 Anatomy of the bifurcation of the carotid artery (from RSN, by permission)

Specimen

A cyst lined by lymphoid tissue.

Pre-operative consideration

The correct diagnosis is the most important consideration. Some branchial cysts are solid and the differentiation from a lymph node may be difficult. It is important in these instances to exclude a primary carcinoma of the head and neck by panendoscopy of the upper respiratory and gastrointestinal tracts. Occasionally a branchial cyst may transmit carotid pulsation, but is never in itself pulsatile. A high branchial cyst may be indistinguishable from a parotid tumour.

Risks

1. Haematoma.
2. Failure to remove the entire cyst with subsequent recurrence.
3. Damage to nerves:
   - Greater auricular nerve.
   - Accessory nerve.
   - Hypoglossal nerve.
   - Mandibular division of the facial nerve (injudiciously placed incision or from excessive elevation of the upper flap).
   - Vagus nerve (close to the carotid sheath).

Preparation

General anaesthesia delivered through an endotracheal tube. The patient is supine on the table, with the neck extended by a small pillow under the shoulders, the head turned to the opposite side from the cyst and stabilized on a head ring.

Method

1. Figure 20.10 shows the approximate typical position of a branchial cyst. A horizontal incision, in a skin crease, at the level of the cyst, is marked out. This incision is deepened through the platysmal layers and the skin flaps elevated superiorly and inferiorly in the subplatysmal plane.
2. The cyst typically lies at the anterior border of the sternomastoid. The external jugular vein lying on the sternomastoid muscle may require to be divided and ligated. The cyst should be freed medially from the anterior border of the sternomastoid by dividing the layer of deep cervical fascia along the anterior border of the muscle. Care should be taken to avoid damaging the greater auricular nerve during this manoeuvre. The cyst is freed from the sternomastoid with dissection as close to the cyst wall as is

possible. Posteriorly as the dissection deepens the accessory nerve can potentially be damaged.

3. With progressive gauze and sharp dissection the cyst is progressively freed. Anteriorly the posterior facial vein may have to be divided and ligated.

4. Superiorly the cyst is freed from the posterior belly of the digastric muscle and it is important that the deeper lying hypoglossal nerve should be identified and preserved. Rarely a branchial cyst may have a connection to the pharynx and in this circumstance the connection passes between the internal and external carotid arteries superior to the hypoglossal nerve.

5. Finally the cyst is removed from the carotid sheath. With haemostasis secure, a suction drain is inserted and the wounds closed in two layers.

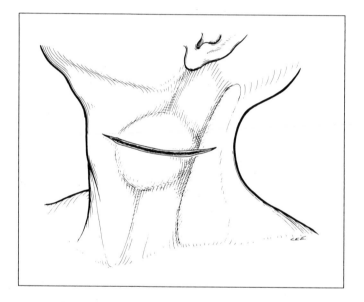

Figure 20.10   Typical site of a branchial cyst (from RSN, by permission)

Post-operative care

The drain is removed when there is a minimum of drainage.

SURGERY FOR PHARYNGEAL POUCH

Indications

There is debate as to the correct treatment of a pharyngeal pouch. If a pouch is small and causing minimal symptoms, particularly in an elderly or frail patient, then no surgery may be appropriate. In patients who have severe dysphagia, regurgitation, cough and chest infection, as a result of overspill surgical intervention is preferable. There are advocates for Dohlmann's procedure, which is described under the endoscopic surgery section (Chapter 19, page 252).

External approach surgery may involve excision, inversion, plication, suspension or a mixture of these various techniques in the management of the pharyngeal pouch. It is preferable for the surgeon to have a flexible approach and to choose a particular technique to fit the needs of an individual patient.

In this section we will describe external pouch surgery up to the location and dissection of the pouch and then consider some of the variations in the management of the pouch.

Pre-operative considerations

If the patient is debilitated, dehydrated or has an overspill chest infection then these factors should be corrected prior to the surgery. Active chest physiotherapy is helpful. When the pouch is large it may be necessary to wash out the pouch prior to operation.

Risks

1. Haematoma.
2. Surgical emphysema. This resolves spontaneously.
3. Fistula with salivary leak. This will eventually heal spontaneously and feeding through the nasogastric tube should continue until this occurs.
4. Vocal cord paralysis from damage to the left recurrent nerve.
5. Infection, either locally or extending into the mediastinum, is usually prevented by antibiotic cover.
6. Pouch recurrence. The division of the cricopharyngeus is believed to reduce the incidence of recurrence.
7. Pharyngeal stenosis can occur and may relate either to excessive tightness in the pharyngeal repair or the lack of a cricopharyngeal myotomy.
8. It is important to realize that a patient's normal swallowing mechanism may take a few months before it returns to what the patient considers normal.

Preparation

A general anaesthetic is provided through a cuffed endotracheal tube. The patient lies supine with a pillow or sandbag under the shoulders to extend the neck. As the surgical approach to the pouch is generally from the left side the chin is turned to the right (opposite side) with the head placed on a head ring. The patient receives an injection of a broad spectrum antibiotic at the time of induction of the anaesthesia.

Method

1. Initial direct endoscopic examination of the pouch is important to exclude the presence of a carcinoma within the pouch. The entrance to the pouch lies posterior to the entrance to the oesophagus. Scopes and instruments typically enter easily into the pouch. The pouch is sucked out through the pharyngoscope and then packed with flavine ribbon gauze. A nasogastric tube is inserted through the nose and guided into the oesophagus.
2. A vertical incision along the anterior margin of the left sternomastoid muscle centred at the level of the cricoid cartilage gives good access. Care has to be taken not to damage the greater auricular nerve at the upper end of the incision. Some operators use a transverse skin crease incision at the level of the cricoid cartilage. The access from this incision in dealing with large pouches can sometimes be limited.
3. The incision is deepened through platysma and then the cervical fascia along the anterior border of the sternomastoid is divided, allowing the sternomastoid muscle to be retracted laterally and revealing the sterno-hyoid, sternothyroid and omohyoid muscles.
4. The omohyoid muscle is divided and a plane of dissection created between the sternomastoid muscle and great vessels laterally and the larynx, trachea and thyroid gland medially. The middle thyroid vein usually requires to be ligated and divided to permit the thyroid gland to be retracted medially.

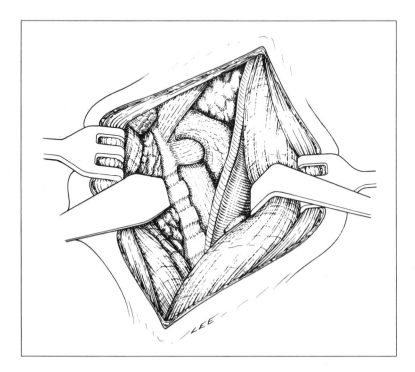

Figure 20.11   Identification of the neck of the pharyngeal pouch. Note its relation to the horizontal fibres of cricopharyngeus (from RSN, by permission)

5. Figure 20.11 shows the sternomastoid and great vessels retracted laterally
    while the trachea and thyroid gland are retracted medially. The pouch is
    identified anterior to the cervical spine, posterior to the thyroid gland,
    trachea and oesophagus. The nasogastric tube allows easy identification of
    the oesophagus. The pouch is grasped with gentle tissue holding forceps
    and cleaned by blunt dissection to expose the neck where it enters into the
    pharynx.

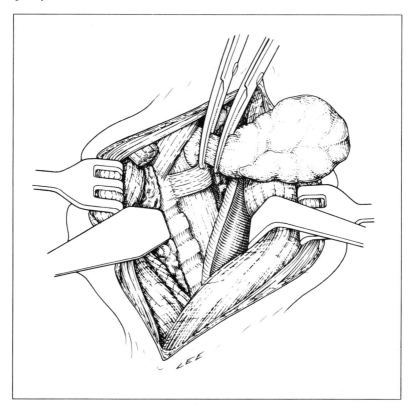

Figure 20.12   Removal of the pouch

6. It is at this point that surgeons differ widely in their technique:
    *   Removal. To remove the pouch, two pairs of forceps are applied across
        the neck (as shown in Figure 20.12). Curved artery forceps or the
        Satinsky clamp, as used in vascular surgery, are satisfactory for this
        purpose. It is important that the most proximal artery clip is not tight
        against the oesophagus as this may predispose to a stricture in this area
        after the closure has been effected. Ribbon gauze packing is removed
        from the pouch prior to operating on the pouch itself. The pouch is
        divided between the forceps and removed. A continuous 2-0 chromic
        catgut is applied over the proximal remaining forceps and tightened as
        the forceps are withdrawn. The space in the muscle of the pharyngeal
        wall through which the pouch protuded is now repaired with inter-
        rupted absorbable sutures.

- Inversion. As an alternative to excision of the pouch some surgeons invert the pouch into the oesophagus and then oversew the gap in the pharyngeal wall through which the pouch protruded.
- Plication. A non-absorbable suture can be used to plicate the pouch and prevent food from entering the pouch.
- Suspension. Another choice is to plicate the pouch partly and suspend the apex of the pouch above the pharyngeal entrance into the pouch.

7. Once surgery has been performed on the pouch most surgeons would advocate a cricopharyngeal myotomy. This is discussed in more detail on page 280. The fibres of cricopharyngeus are located inferior to the repaired site of the neck of the pouch. These fibres are carefully divided down to the oesophageal mucosa with a scalpel. The use of an operating microscope often facilitates accurate muscle division. Figure 20.13 demonstrates the myotomy.

8. With haemostasis secure a suction drain is inserted. The wound is closed in two layers with absorbable sutures to platysma and then either non-absorbable sutures or clips to the skin.

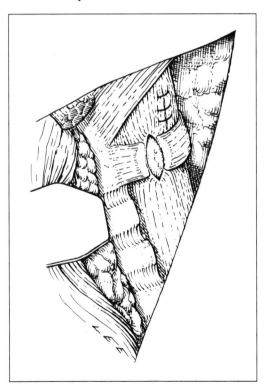

Figure 20.13 The horizontal fibres of cricopharyngeus have been divided (from RSN, by permission)

Post-operative care

Antibiotic cover should continue for approximately 7 days. The suction drain is removed when there is minimal drainage (less than 10 ml in 24 hours), which usually occurs after about 48 hours. The patient is fed through the nasogastric tube for between 5 and 7 days whenever a pouch is excised or when there is any breach (or suspicion of breach) of the oesophagus.

CRICOPHARYNGEAL SPHINCTEROTOMY

Indications

1. Motor neurone disease with the onset of progressive dysphagia. Early surgery is helpful, particularly if the patient complains of spill-over into the larynx. There should be reasonable tongue mobility to allow some success from this operation.
2. The pharyngeal paralysis arising from a brain stem cerebrovascular accident or from lesions high in the vagus.
3. The rare form of ocular pharyngeal muscular dystrophy.
4. Small pharyngeal pouches and inco-ordination of the upper oesophageal sphincter.
5. A sphincterotomy is a necessary part of a supraglottic laryngectomy to improve swallowing.

Pre-operative considerations

A cricopharyngeal sphincterotomy may exacerbate gastro-oesophageal reflux. If the patient has a neuromuscular disorder pre-operative liaison with the anaesthetist is important to allow the correct choice of anaesthetic agents and technique.

Method

1. The surgical approach to a cricopharyngeal sphincterotomy is as for the approach to a pharyngeal pouch. (See page 275.) The sphincterotomy is optimally carried out with the use of the operating microscope. Figure 22.14 demonstrates the anatomical position for a cricopharyngeal sphincterotomy. It is useful to have a bronchoscope, a large oesophageal bougie or a partially inflated Foley catheter within the oesophagus to place the cricopharyngeus muscle on the stretch.
2. A sphincterotomy of between 4 and 5 cm is created as close to the posterior mid-line as possible to avoid injuring the recurrent laryngeal nerve. The incision should extend inferiorly into the upper muscles of the oesophagus and superiorly into the inferior pharyngeal constrictor. The oesophageal mucosa should be able to bulge throughout the length of the myotomy. Close inspection of the mucosa is required to ensure that it has not been perforated.

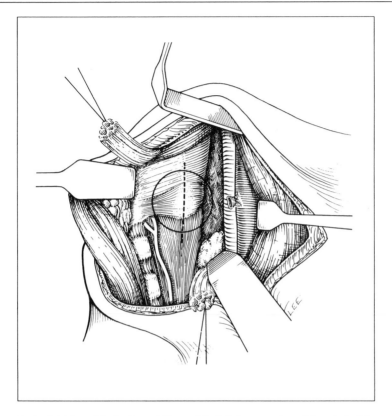

Figure 20.14 Division of the horizontal fibres of the inferior constrictor. Note the incision extends into the longitudinal fibres of the oesophagus (from RSN, by permission)

Post-operative care and specific complications

1. These are essentially as for external treatment of a pharyngeal pouch (see page 279).
2. Failure to divide the cricopharyngeus will result in failure of the operation.
3. Massive tracheobronchial aspiration can occur.

Chapter 21

Surgery of the larynx

LARYNGOFISSURE

Introduction

Laryngofissure is a surgical approach to the larynx. The indication for a laryngofissure will depend on the pathology within the larynx. A laryngofissure may be used for access to treat:

1. A laryngocoele.
2. To confirm the nature of intralaryngeal pathology and to obtain a biopsy.
3. As a preliminary to treatment of squamous cell carcinoma of the vocal cords by vertical hemilaryngectomy.
4. To treat intralaryngeal trauma and to stabilize fractures of the thyroid cartilage.

Specimen

This will depend on the pathology.

Pre-operative considerations

The advent of the more advanced radiological investigations has reduced the need for laryngofissure.

Should a vertical partial laryngectomy be planned then it is important that the patient is also consented for a total laryngectomy in case tumour is outwith the safe margins for a partial laryngectomy.

A temporary tracheostomy must always be performed at the time of laryngofissure and therefore the patient should be forewarned that he or she will not be able to speak immediately after the procedure.

Risks

These are largely dependent on the pathology for which laryngofissure was performed and include:

1. Persistent mild dysphonia.
2. Intralaryngeal adhesions.
3. Failure to treat the pathology fully for which the laryngofissure was performed.

Preparation

The operation commences with general oral endotracheal anaesthesia. The patient is supine on the table with a sand bag under the shoulder to extend the neck and a head ring to support the head. The first procedure is to perform the tracheostomy and then anaesthesia should continue via the tracheostomy tube. Tracheostomy is discussed in Chapter 20, page 258.

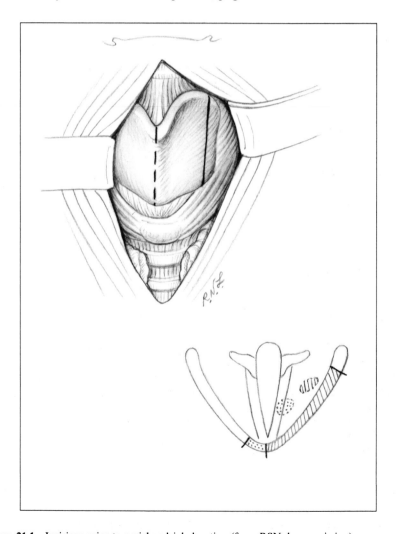

Figure 21.1 Incisions prior to perichondrial elevation (from RSN, by permission)

Method

1. A horizontal or collar incision centred over the Adam's apple of the thyroid cartilage is deepened through the platysma to the strap muscles overlying the thyroid cartilage. These strap muscles are parted in the mid-line and then reflected laterally.
2. A vertical incision is made in the mid-line of the thyroid cartilage, firstly through the external perichondrium, secondly through the thyroid cartilage, and thirdly through the internal layer of perichondrium. It is then possible to retract both alae of the thyroid cartilage laterally to allow direct inspection of the laryngeal lumen.
3. The incision through the perichondrium and cartilage may vary, depending on the precise intralaryngeal pathology. For example, in a vertical partial laryngectomy, the perichondrium on the external surface of the thyroid cartilage may first be peeled from the cartilage and then the cartilage itself resected with the affected portion of the vocal cord. Figure 21.1 demonstrates with vertical lines the area where the perichondrium is elevated and the cartilage subsequently divided prior to removal of the affected vocal cord during a vertical partial laryngectomy. In other instances, for example fracture of the thyroid cartilage in combination with intralaryngeal injuries, the precise nature of the incision will alter.

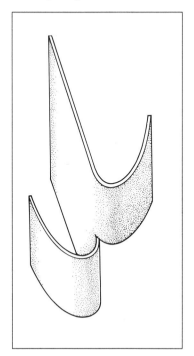

Figure 21.2 A silastic keel (from RSN, by permission)

4. When there is a risk that laryngeal stenosis may follow the intralaryngeal surgery from a laryngofissure a stent should be inserted. This may take the form of a silastic keel, such as that shown in Figure 21.2. This keel is

inserted between the lamina of the thyroid cartilage and sutured to the thyroid lamina using 3-0 chromic catgut, as demonstrated in Figure 21.3. Such a stent is removed endoscopically 6 weeks later, when gentle traction on the silastic will tear loose the absorbable stay sutures.

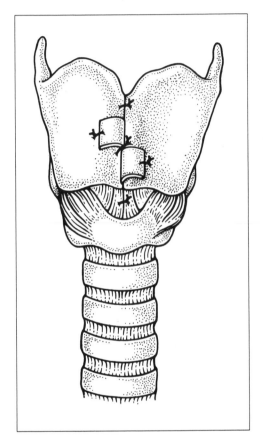

Figure 21.3 The keel sutured in position (from RSN, by permission)

5. To close, the external perichondrial layers of the thyroid cartilage are sutured together with absorbable sutures. The strap muscles are re-opposed in the mid-line and then the cutaneous wound is closed, first with chromic catgut to the platysmal layer and then non-absorbable sutures or staples to skin.

Post-operative care

When there has not been extensive mucosal damage within the larynx and a stent has not been required then the tracheostomy can be corked from about day 2 and removed after 3–4 days. The subsequent management will depend on the intralaryngeal pathology.

If a stent has been inserted than the tracheostomy must remain *in situ* until the stent is removed endoscopically after 6 weeks.

TOTAL LARYNGECTOMY

Indications

1. Squamous carcinoma of the larynx
   - failed radiotherapy
   - transglottic tumours
   - T3 glottic tumours (? males)
   - T3 and T4 supraglottic tumours
   - post-cricoid tumours (part of the resection)
   - laryngeal radionecrosis
2. Non-squamous tumours which do not respond to radiotherapy.
3. Intractable aspiration (e.g. in motor neurone disease).
4. Laryngeal papillomata (very rarely).

Specimen

Larynx, thyroid cartilage, cricoid cartilage, epiglottis, hyoid bone, strap muscles, one or two lobes of thyroid gland.

Pre-operative considerations

Preparation begins the week before surgery, to include meeting a laryngectomized patient and to receive counselling from medical, nursing, physiotherapy and speech therapy staff. Baseline measures of biochemical and haematological parameters should be made. Cross matched blood should be arranged.

An antibiotic which covers both aerobic and anaerobic organisms may be given with the anaesthetic pre-medication and continued for 48 hours postoperatively.

Risks

1. Local wound problems.
2. Tracheostomy problems, such as excessive secretions.
3. Temporary paralytic ileus.
4. Hypocalcaemia.
5. Hypothyroidism.
6. Pharyngeal stenosis.
7. Pharyngocutaneous fistula.
8. Failure to obtain an 'oesophageal' voice.

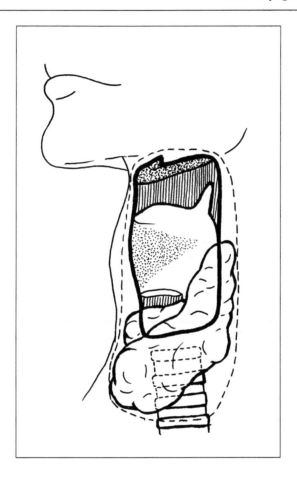

Figure 21.4 The solid line illustrates the total laryngectomy specimen, plus a variable amount of upper trachea. The dotted line shows the pharyngolaryngo-oesophagectomy specimen to include total laryngectomy specimen, thyroid gland and pharynx with a portion of upper oesophagus

Preparation

General anaesthetic is delivered through an oral endotracheal tube. When the tumour is large and severely compromises both airway and endotracheal intubation then a preliminary tracheostomy under local anaesthetic should be performed. This tracheostomy can be performed a couple of days before or at the time of laryngectomy and it should be performed 'high' and the tract excised at the time of definitive operation.

The patient is placed supine on the table (tilted foot-down), neck extended.

Incisions

1. A 'U'-shaped incision (modified Gluck Sorensen) which commences on

each side at the anterior border of the sternomastoid at the level of the hyoid bone and curves downwards to meet immediately below the cricoid cartilage. This is usually satisfactory even in post-radiotherapy cases.

2. A vertical incision is classically used to treat radionecrosis. The pharyngeal repair and skin incision lie in the same line which is undesirable.

3. A half 'H' incision when a neck dissection is combined with the laryngectomy.

4. When a radical neck dissection is performed with a laryngectomy following radiotherapy the operation may be performed either through extensions of the double McFee incision or the vertical limb of a half 'H' can be sited along the anterior margin of the trapezius.

Stoma siting

The stoma can be sited either in the lower flap or in the wound.

Method

1. A 'U' incision is performed. Flaps are elevated in the subplatysmal plane. The limit to the upper flap is when the hyoid bone can be freely palpated and the suprahyoid muscles are visible. This flap is anchored to the head towels with sutures placed in the subcutaneous tissues. Lower flap dissection depends on access and the position for the stoma.

2. The mid-line structures of the neck (larynx, strap muscles and thyroid gland) are separated from the lateral structures (carotid sheath and sternomastoid). On both sides the fascia along the anterior border of sternomastoid is incised, the omohyoid where it crosses the carotid sheath is divided and the middle thyroid veins are divided and ligated. The superior laryngeal pedicle is separated by blunt dissection and the superior thyroid artery is suture ligated, internal laryngeal nerve divided and the superior thyroid veins ligated and divided. On the side of the tumour (the side of thyroid lobe sacrifice) the inferior thyroid artery is double ligated and divided.

3. The sternohyoid and sternothyroid muscles are divided above the sternum. The trachea is exposed in the mid-line and the inferior thyroid veins which run close to the trachea are isolated, divided and ligated. On the side of thyroid lobe preservation the strap muscles are peeled upwards from the surface of the gland, the isthmus of the gland is divided and then the lobe to be preserved is peeled away laterally from the trachea. This is shown in Figure 21.5.

4. The hyoid bone is mobilized. The suprahyoid muscles (genioglossus, hypoglossus, mylohyoid, the digastric sling and middle constrictor) are separated by subperiosteal dissection. The tip of the greater horn has to be dissected out close to the bone as the lingual artery lies directly superior and it is at risk.

5. The posterior margins of the thyroid cartilage can now be skeletonized as shown in Figure 21.6. Note the divided superior laryngeal pedicle. A scalpel divides the fibres of the inferior constrictor in a vertical direction

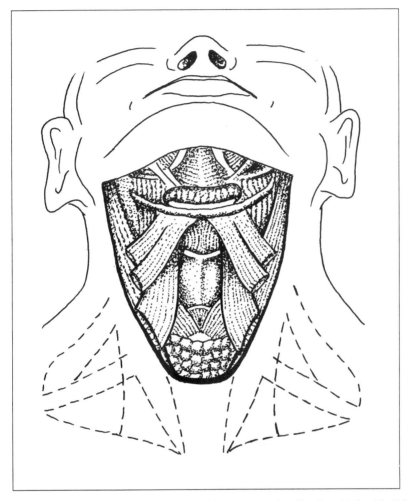

Figure 21.5 Exposure of the larynx. Division of the strap muscles. The thyroid gland is divided next

just anterior to the posterior margin of the thyroid cartilage. Subperiosteal reflection posteriorly preserves the muscle and periosteum for pharyngeal reconstruction. Tissue preservation should only be performed with due consideration to the site and size of the tumour.

6. The trachea can be divided at this point. If the stoma is to be through the lower flap a 2 × 2 cm hole is cut in the flap. Stout stay sutures of silk are placed through the skin, the peritracheal fascia (not penetrating the tracheal mucosa) and back through the skin. The tracheal division is bevelled – low at the front, higher at the back – to facilitate a flush surface when the trachea is rotated into its final position. A ribbon gauze is placed in the lower end of the specimen to obstruct laryngeal secretions and a cuffed 'tracheostomy type' anaesthetic tube is inserted.

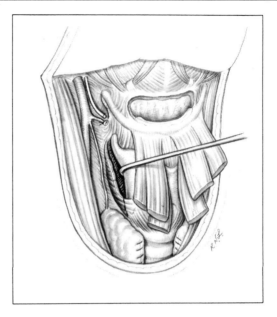

Figure 21.6   Identification of the posterior border of thyroid cartilage (from RSN, by permission)

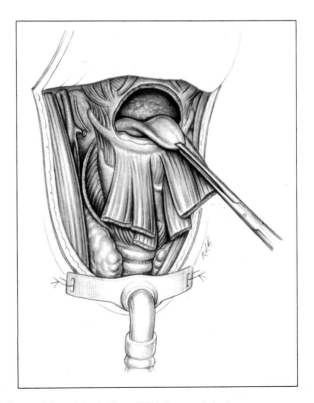

Figure 21.7   Delivery of the epiglottis (from RSN, by permission)

7. The pharynx is opened from the side opposite the tumour. There is danger in dissecting inferiorly behind the hyoid bone and entering the pre-epiglottic space. The epiglottis may be palpable prior to opening the pharynx. The epiglottis is grasped in a pair of Allis forceps and pulled forwards. This is shown in Figure 21.7.

8. The pharyngeal mucosa is divided on the side away from the tumour, first by aiming at the superior cornu of the thyroid cartilage on that side. This allows the tumour to be seen and the excision margins to be planned. In general the cut on the side of the tumour is towards the superior cornu of the thyroid cartilage and then the cuts are close to the margins of the thyroid ala on both sides. The horizontal cut is at the level of the cricoarytenoid joint and a finger inserted into the upper oesophagus prevents the oesophagus being damaged as the specimen is being separated from the oesophagus. This tumour removal and the bevel of the trachea to form the tracheostomy are shown in Figure 21.8.

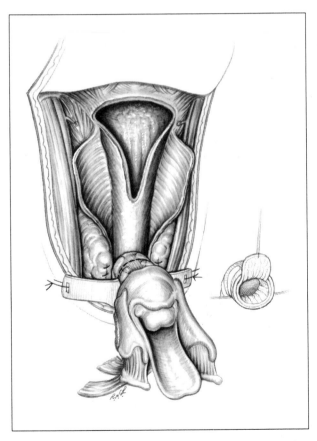

Figure 21.8 Dissection of the larynx from the hypopharynx and cervical oesophagus (from RSN, by permission)

9.   The surgical team changes gown, gloves and instruments and the wound is
     washed out with sterile water. A nasogastric tube is inserted from the
     nose.
10. Pharyngeal closure is in three layers with absorbable sutures. The first
     layer may be interrupted or an inverting continuous suture. Depending on
     the defect, this layer may be a straight line or in the shape of a T. The
     second layer reinforces the first while the third layer gently apposes the
     pharyngeal muscles. One form of closure is shown in Figure 21.9. Note
     that in this illustration both lobes of thyroid have been preserved.

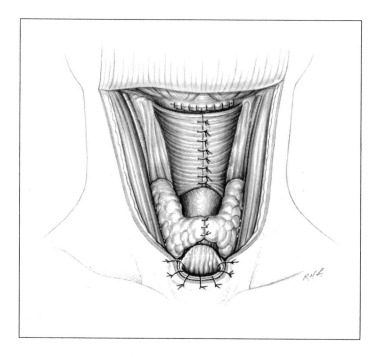

Figure 21.9   Closure following laryngectomy (from RSN, by permission)

11. Two layers are required to fashion the tracheostomy – the peritracheal
     fascia is stitched to the platysmal layer and then the tracheal mucosa is
     apposed to the skin with a non-absorbable suture.
12. Haemostasis is checked in the wound and two suction drains are inserted,
     one each to the gutters of the neck. Care is taken that the drains do not
     suck on the great vessels or the pharyngeal repair. Wound closure is in
     two layers – the first is an absorbable suture to the platysmal layer and the
     second a non-absorbable cutaneous closure.

Post-operative

1.   Antibiotics should be given for 2–7 days.

2. Nasogastric feeding for 5–14 days depending on the condition of the tissues (longer interval for radiotherapy cases).
3. The nasogastric feeding should be built up gradually. Loose bowel motions can sometimes be a problem.
4. A contrast radiograph can be performed to confirm the integrity of the pharyngeal closure prior to commencing oral fluids.

VOICE RESTORATION FOLLOWING LARYNGECTOMY

Introduction

The main techniques of producing voice following a total laryngectomy are:

1. An electronic vibrator (electronic larynx), which can be applied to the skin of the patient's neck, to provide sound which he or she vocalizes. This is shown in Figure 21.10.

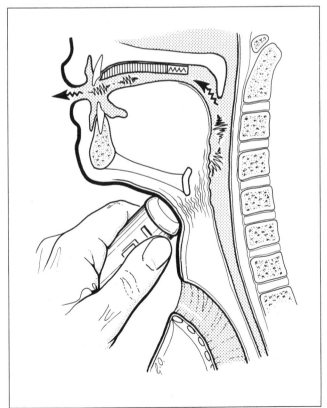

Figure 21.10   Using electronic vibrator to produce sound within the hypopharynx (from RSN, by permission)

2. Oesophageal voice. This is shown in Figure 21.11.
3. Tracheo-oesophageal shunt voice.

We shall now describe the creation of a tracheo-oesophageal fistula and the insertion of the one-way valve prosthesis following total laryngectomy. Figure 21.12 demonstrates the way in which the one-way valved prosthesis helps the patient to phonate. The pharyngeal segment vibrates with the passage of the air. The patient has to occlude the tracheal stoma to facilitate the passage of the air through the one-way valve into the upper oesophagus.

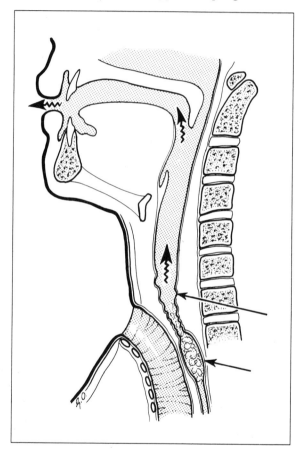

Figure 21.11 Production of oesophageal voice (from RSN, by permission)

Indications

Some surgeons insert a valve at the time of total laryngectomy, whereas most surgeons would recommend a wait of at least 6 months following laryngectomy to permit the patient time to learn oesophageal speech. The insertion of a valve can either be to improve the patient who has oesophageal speech or to help a patient who has failed to learn oesophageal speech.

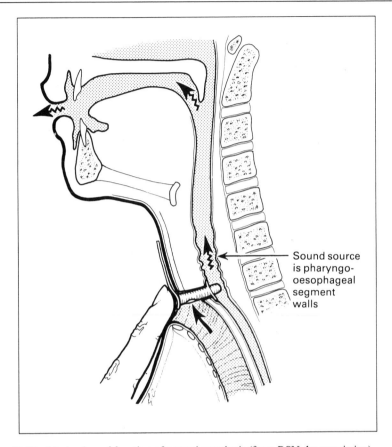

Figure 21.12   Mechanism of function of a vocal prosthesis (from RSN, by permission)

Pre-operative considerations

The patient should have a good tracheal stoma and should be assessed by the surgeon and the speech therapist prior to surgery. Some units use video fluoroscopy to identify the vibrating pharyngo-oesophageal section. It can sometimes be necessary to perform a cricopharyngeal myotomy to facilitate the development of a pharyngo-oesophageal segment. It can also be useful to perform the Taub test prior to insertion of a valve.

Risks

The complications vary, dependent on the type of prosthesis and the skill of fitment:

1. Too long a prosthesis may impinge on the posterior oesophageal wall and cause pain.
2. A short prosthesis may fail to keep the fistula patent.

3. The patient may fail to clean the prosthesis effectively, resulting in blockage.
4. The fistula may close if the prosthesis is left out for too long.
5. The patient may drop the prosthesis down the trachea while attempting reinsertion.
6. Leakage may occur around the fistula.
7. Granulations or bleeding may occur around the fistula.
8. The prosthesis may not fit well because the initial puncture has either been made in the wrong site (too deep within the stoma) or the tracheal stoma has been too narrow to allow proper manipulation and insertion of the prosthesis.

Preparation

In most patients this technique is performed under general anaesthesia delivered through the endotracheal stoma. The patient is supine on the table with a sandbag under the shoulders and a head ring to support the head.

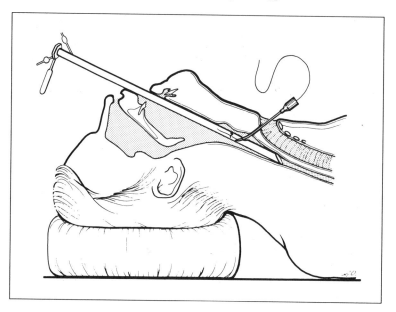

Figure 21.13   Method of fistula creation to fit a vocal prosthesis (from RSN, by permission)

Method

1. A modified bronchoscope or Yankauer sucker, as shown in Figure 21.13, is passed and its distal end or specifically designed hole is palpated through the tracheal stoma to ensure that it is in the correct position. The puncture is planned approximately 5 mm inside the upper mucocutaneous junction of the tracheostome.

2. The puncture is created with a cannula which has silk thread attached. This is led through the mouth and an attached 14 French rubber catheter follows. The catheter is then led distally down into the oesophagus as in Figure 21.14. The catheter is left in place beteeen 2 and 4 days, and at the end of this time the catheter is removed and the prosthesis is inserted.
3. There are a number of different instruments which facilitate the insertion of the different valves. An operator should always consult the manual which is provided by the maker of the valves prior to insertion.

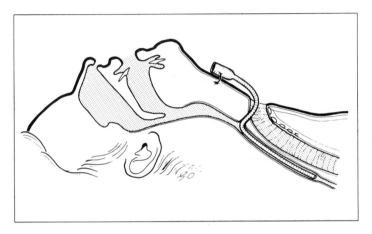

Figure 21.14 Positioning the catheter within the oesophagus in order to create a permanent tracheo-oesophageal fistula (from RSN, by permission)

Post-operative care

In some patients speech improvement is almost immediate. To speak, the patient simply exhales while covering the tracheostome such that pulmonary air enters the pharyngo-oesophageal segments through the prosthesis. The patient is able to talk for longer bursts by this technique compared with normal oesophageal voice.

PHARYNGOLARYNGO-OESOPHAGECTOMY

Indications

This operation is indicated for tumours of the pharynx and cervical oesophagus which directly involve upper thoracic oesophagus, or those tumours whose lower margin prevents adequate resection and repair through the neck alone. This implies tumours of the post-cricoid and upper cervical oesophagus.

Specimen

This usually includes larynx, both lobes of thyroid gland, the pharynx and usually – because one cannot determine the lower limit of the tumour – the oesophagus.

Pre-operative considerations

This is a very major operation and in many patients, particularly the elderly, their general condition may be judged unsuitable for ultra-radical surgery. It is crucial when considering such an operation that metastatic disease or local extension, particularly into the prevertebral muscles which would render the patient incurable, is identified prior to surgery. CT and MR scanning of the neck is useful for identifying prevertebral muscle invasion. Sometimes, however, such evidence of spread of disease may only be discovered at exploration of the neck.

Patients with lower pharyngeal and upper oesophageal lesions often have problems with nutrition and it is important that, pre-operatively, the nutritional status of the patient is carefully considered. The patient may require supplements of calories, proteins and vitamins, given as nutritionally balanced high calorie drinks either orally or via a fine bore nasogastric tube. Parenteral nutrition through an intravenous line may occasionally be required. The creation of a gastrostomy or jejunostomy should be avoided in the preliminary phase as this will contaminate the abdominal field and complicate the work of the abdominal surgical team.

Whenever a radical resection of the pharynx, larynx and oesophagus is contemplated a general surgeon should be involved so that the repair can be planned. Depending on whether the surgeon plans to use a gastric pull-up, a segment of colon, or a jejunal free graft, will determine the required type of bowel preparation. In general, a low residue, high calorie, high vitamin diet to allow a lower residue in the colon with the addition of other medicinal agents to achieve a clean and empty bowel prior to the surgery is useful.

Per-operative antibiotics will be required.

Risks

Neck

1. Haematoma.
2. Abscess formation.
3. Anastomotic breakdown.
4. Fistula.
5. Septicaemic shock.
6. Late anastomotic stenosis.

Chest

7. Pneumothorax.

8.   Mediastinal haemorrhage/haematoma.
9.   Mediastinitis.

Intra-abdominal problems

10.   Intra-abdominal anastomotic leaks.
11.   Paralytic ileus.
12.   Intestinal obstruction.

Endocrine and metabolic

13.   Hypoparathyroidism.
14.   Hypothyroidism.
15.   Electrolyte disturbance.
16.   Renal failure.

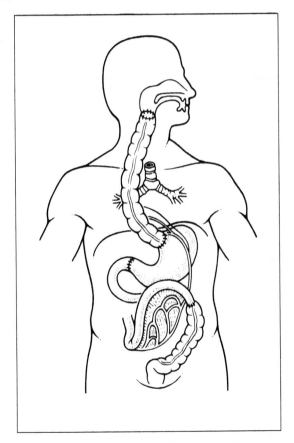

Figure 21.15   Reconstruction using colon (from RSN, by permission)

Preparation

The operation commences with general peroral endotracheal anaesthesia and at a later stage changes to general anaesthesia through a tracheostomy tube. The patient is supine on the table with a sandbag under the shoulder and a head ring under the head to stabilize. The patient is prepared from the mouth to just above the groin and then towels are placed to allow each separate part of the operation to proceed in tandem.

Method

1. The neck incision will depend on precisely what is planned within the neck, but a shallow 'U'-shaped incision is often appropriate. This incision can be extended to include a neck dissection if required.
2. The first part of the neck surgery is to determine the approximate limits of the primary lesion and to confirm that it is resectable. Any suspicious lymph nodes should be removed and sent for frozen section review.
3. The neck procedure is essentially a total laryngectomy and pharyngectomy with the addition of a total thyroidectomy. The paratracheal and para-oesophageal areolar and lymphatic tissue is removed with the specimen and often a radical neck dissection is required. Any neck dissection specimen and the cervical visual specimen is left transected below the larynx and a cuffed tracheostomy tube is inserted.
4. A general surgeon opens the abdomen and prepares the part of the bowel which is to replace the pharynx and oesophagus. The oesophagus is mobilized from below by finger dissection and then the entire specimen, which includes the larynx and pharynx and oesophagus, is removed through the neck.
5. Figure 21.15 demonstrates a segment of colon interposed to replace pharynx and oesophagus, whereas Figure 21.16 demonstrates the use of a gastric pull-up.
6. Closure-suction drains are always required in the neck and chest drains are often inserted electively. The neck wound is closed in two layers and the tracheostome fashioned as for the total laryngectomy.

Post-operative care

The neck part of the procedure is managed as for a total laryngectomy. The drains are removed when there is less than 10 ml drainage in the previous 24 hours.

The nasogastric feeding can often be delayed compared with a total laryngectomy as a result of the intra-abdominal surgery. Nasograstric feeding commences when bowel sounds return to normal. Alternatively, the general surgeon may have created a temporary feeding jejunostomy and, in this case, feeding is through the tube, when bowel sounds and evidence of normal bowel function have returned.

Careful monitoring of serum calcium and its appropriate replacement is essential as both thyroid lobes, including parathyroid glands, have been removed. The advice of an endocrinologist concerning long-term replacement is also useful. The patient will require regular thyroid supplements, plus some form of calcium supplements.

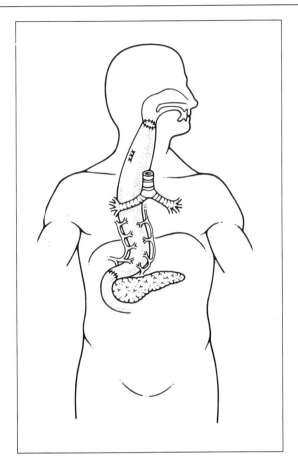

Figure 21.16 Reconstruction using the 'gastric pull-up technique' (from RSN, by permission)

Close monitoring of the chest is required. Chest infection and pulmonary collapse is a danger and should be intensively treated with regular physiotherapy.

Colonic transpositions passed through the short anterior or retrosternal route are less liable to intrathoracic problems. The longer posterior route for a gastric pull-up gives a considerable risk of mediastinal haemorrhage, haematoma or infection and these must be actively searched for and treated as appropriate. If chest drains have been inserted then these can be removed when there is no evidence of a pneumothorax. If chest drains have not been inserted then very close observation is required to ensure that the patient does not develop a pneumothorax.

The commonest site of breakdown for both the gastric pull-ups and colonic interpositions is at the pharyngocolic or pharyngogastric junction. Close observation should be made for this potentially lethal problem.

Post-operative voice following the transpositions can be quite variable. A number of patients have developed colonic or gastric speech.

Chapter 22

Neck dissection

Squamous carcinoma of the head and neck metastasize typically to the lymph nodes in the neck. These nodes form a line of defence prior to systemic dissemination. The inferior end of the internal jugular vein is the exit point from this barrier. Management of nodal disease is dependent on the primary site and its treatment requirements, TNM/AJC classification and general patient condition, in addition to local radiotherapy facilities and philosophies.

A number of types of neck dissections have been described.

1. Radical neck dissection (described below)

Clearance of lymph-bearing tissue in the neck between the skull base and mandible superiorly, clavicle inferiorly, the mid-line of the neck and the anterior border of the trapezius muscle.

The specimen contains sternocleidomastoid, internal jugular vein, submandibular gland and tail of parotid. The accessory nerve is divided.

2. Functional neck dissection

This dissection differs from the radical dissection in that any or all of the following structures may be conserved: sternomastoid, internal jugular vein and accessory nerve.

3. Block dissection

One specific region of the neck may be removed, i.e. suprahyoid block dissection.

Pre-operative considerations

The radical neck dissection is the 'gold standard' operation in the surgical management of neck lymph node metastasis from squamous carcinoma. The following description will concentrate on that procedure.

It is important to be fully conversant with the relevant neck anatomy prior to undertaking a radical neck dissection.

Risks

1. Wound haematoma.
2. A chylous leak through the drain. In general this requires an exploration of the lower part of the neck dissection, although on occasion conservative management with pressure may be adequate.
3. Expected nerve deficits include the accessory nerve, and the cutaneous branches to the neck skin. Neck and shoulder stiffness commonly follow accessory nerve division.
4. Potential nerve deficits include lingual branch of 5, mandibular branch of 7, glossopharyngeal, vagus, hypoglossal, phrenic and brachial plexus. The site of the nodal mass will give prior warning of post-operative neurological deficits.
5. Facial oedema, cerebral oedema can develop particularly when the neck dissection is a bilateral procedure. A time interval of at least 6 weeks between the first and second side neck dissections reduces the incidence of post-operative oedema.
6. Excessive scarring and tethering by the neck incisions.
7. Failure to control the disease.

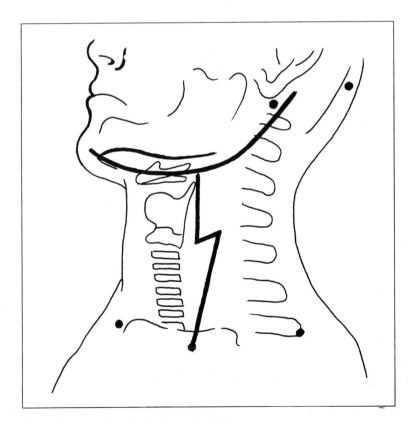

Figure 22.1 Y incision with hitch in descending limb

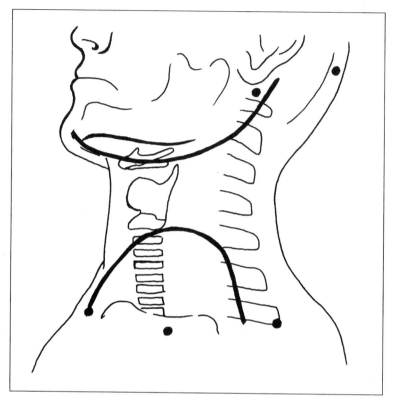

Figure 22.2   Horizontal incisions of McFee

Preparation

General anaesthesia through nasal or oral endotracheal tube. Supine on table, neck extended by sandbag under shoulder, point of chin rotated to the opposite side, head-up tilt to the table.

Incisions

1. Non-irradiated neck (Figure 22.1). Upper incision curved from mastoid to hyoid bone and up to point of chin. Vertical limb, with a lazy 'S' from the mid point of the upper incision to the mid point of the clavicle.
2. Irradiated neck (Figure 22.2). McFee incision. Upper incision as for non-irradiated neck with curved lower incision parallel to the upper incision. The waist should be about 4 cm wide.
3. Previous neck surgery or combined procedures may alter the design of the skin incisions.

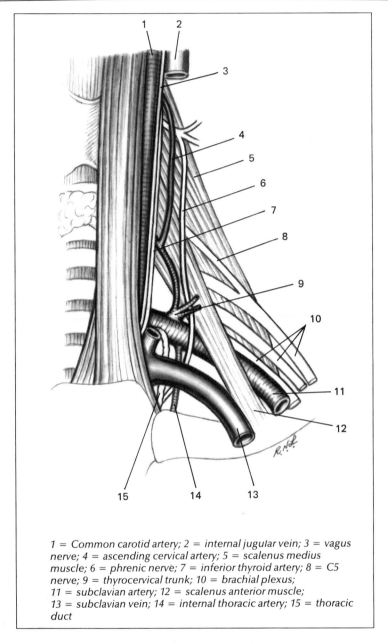

1 = Common carotid artery; 2 = internal jugular vein; 3 = vagus nerve; 4 = ascending cervical artery; 5 = scalenus medius muscle; 6 = phrenic nerve; 7 = inferior thyroid artery; 8 = C5 nerve; 9 = thyrocervical trunk; 10 = brachial plexus; 11 = subclavian artery; 12 = scalenus anterior muscle; 13 = subclavian vein; 14 = internal thoracic artery; 15 = thoracic duct

Figure 22.3 Anatomy of root of neck (from RSN, by permission)

Method

1. Skin flaps are elevated incorporating platysma. The upper flap is raised in a plane deep to the capsule of the submandibular gland to preserve the mandibular division of the facial nerve.

2. The lower end of the sternomastoid is placed under tension and the muscle divided with a knife approximately 2 cm above its clavicular insertion. Bleeding vessels are cauterized during the muscle division. The internal jugular vein, deep to the sternomastoid, lying anterolateral in the carotid sheath, is carefully isolated for a length of 3 cm. Tributaries are isolated, ligated and divided. The vagus nerve lying on the carotid artery is identified and care is taken that this structure is not incorporated in any ligatures. The relevant anatomy is shown in Figure 22.3.

3. Two stout ligatures of silk above and two below are placed around the jugular vein. A suture ligature is placed through the lower end and the internal jugular vein is divided with a knife. Figure 22.4.

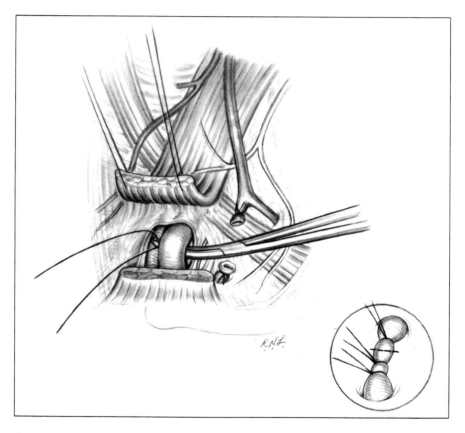

Figure 22.4 Isolation and ligation of lower end internal jugular vein (from RSN, by permission)

4. The supraclavicular triangle is now tackled and the relevant anatomy is shown in Figure 22.5. The omohyoid muscle, lateral to the carotid sheath, is divided. Blunt dissection through the fat pad lateral to the carotid sheath to the fascia over the anterior surface of scalenus anterior allows

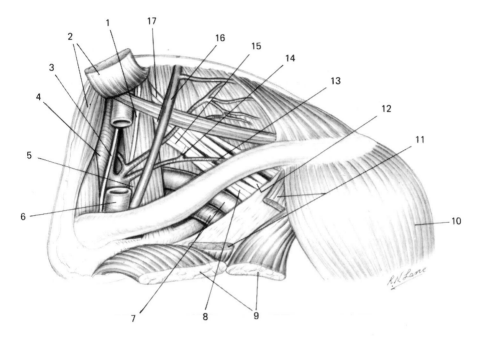

1 = Phrenic nerve; 2 = sternomastoid muscle; 3 = vagus nerve;
4 = common carotid artery; 5 = scalenus anterior muscle;
6 = internal jugular vein; 7 = subclavian artery and vein;
8 = posterior cord of brachial plexus; 9 = pectoralis major
muscle; 10 = deltoid muscle; 11 = pectoralis minor muscle;
12 = lateral cord; 13 = suprascapular artery; 14 = descending
scapular artery; 15 = lower trunk; 16 = external jugular vein;
17 = upper trunk of the brachial plexus

Figure 22.5   Supraclavicular anatomy (from RSN, by permission)

the phrenic nerve running in an inferomedial direction to be identified. A finger is passed laterally between the pre-vertebral fascia and the fat pad to the anterior border of trapezius. The external jugular vein and transverse cervical vessels are ligated and divided before the supraclavicular fat pad is divided by cutting down on to the finger with a knife. This is shown in Figure 22.6. The branchial plexus is deep to the pre-vertebral fascia at this point.

5. A tunnel is formed with the finger along the anterior border of the trapezius up to the sternomastoid between fat and pre-vertebral fascia as shown in Figure 22.7. The fat is divided progressively between heavy artery clips. The accessory nerve is divided during this manoeuvre.

6. Sharp dissection along the line of the vagus nerve allows the jugular vein to be elevated out of the carotid sheath. Care should be taken to ensure that the inferior thyroid artery or its origin from the thyrocervical trunk are not torn during this manoeuvre. The specimen can now be peeled free from the pre-vertebral fascia in an antero-superior direction. Branches of the cervical plexus are divided close to the specimen as it is elevated.

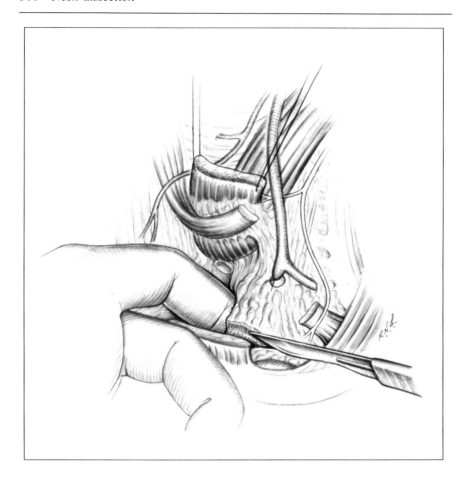

Figure 22.6 Supraclavicular dissection (from RSN, by permission)

7. The anatomy of the upper end of the internal jugular vein is shown in
    Figure 22.8. The posterior belly of digastric is identified and when
    retracted superiorly allows the upper end of the internal jugular vein to be
    identified. Finger dissection from a posterior direction, deep to the upper
    end of sternocleidomastoid onto the transverse process of atlas (C1),
    allows the upper end of sternomastoid to be divided from the mastoid
    process while a finger protects the jugular vein. The internal jugular vein is
    freed over a distance of approximately 2 cm. The occipital artery and vein
    which run parallel to the inferior border of the posterior belly of digastric
    may need ligation and division. Identification of the vagus nerve (between
    jugular vein and internal carotid artery), the accessory nerve (running
    posteriorly superficial to the jugular vein) and the hypoglossal nerve
    (emerging anteriorly between the jugular vein and the internal carotid
    artery) should be made prior to placing two stout silk sutures above and
    one below the vein, which is then ligated and divided. This is shown in
    Figure 22.9.

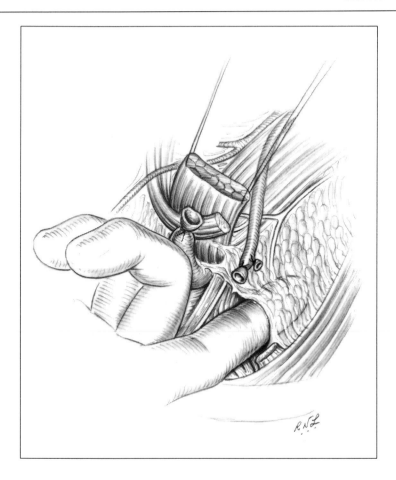

Figure 22.7 Dissection of posterior triangle (from RSN, by permission)

8. The specimen can now be freed from the submandibular triangle. The anatomy of this area is shown in Figure 22.10. The submandibular gland, grasped in forceps, is dissected from its capsule. Ligation and division of the facial artery and common facial vein is at the upper border of the gland. Submental fat and the superficial lobe of the gland are dissected posteriorly and freed from the posterior margin of the mylohyoid muscle. The mylohyoid muscle is retracted forward by a blunt retractor and the gland pulled inferiorly. This demonstrates the lingual nerve which is then separated from the gland and duct in this position. The submandibular duct is ligated as far anterior as is possible.
9. Division of the fascia overlying the suprahyoid strap muscles allows the neck dissection specimen to be removed (Figure 22.11).
10. Gowns, gloves and instruments may be changed. The wound is washed.
11. Haemostasis is secured. The areas to check specifically are the posterior surface of a bridge flap, the lower end of the jugular vein for chylous leaks and the vena commitantes of the hypoglossal nerves.

12. Two suction drains are inserted, avoiding the carotid artery when positioned. The wound is closed in two layers, absorbable sutures to platysma and a cutaneous closure with non-absorbable sutures or clips.

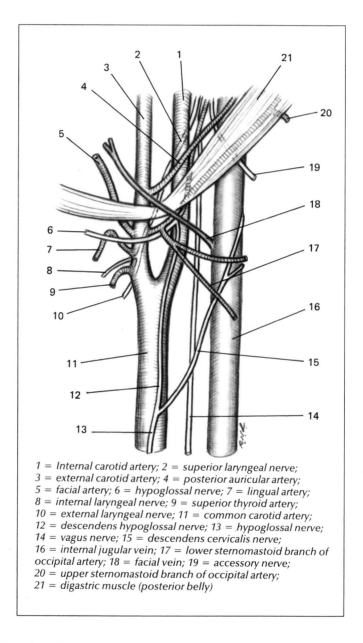

1 = Internal carotid artery; 2 = superior laryngeal nerve;
3 = external carotid artery; 4 = posterior auricular artery;
5 = facial artery; 6 = hypoglossal nerve; 7 = lingual artery;
8 = internal laryngeal nerve; 9 = superior thyroid artery;
10 = external laryngeal nerve; 11 = common carotid artery;
12 = descendens hypoglossal nerve; 13 = hypoglossal nerve;
14 = vagus nerve; 15 = descendens cervicalis nerve;
16 = internal jugular vein; 17 = lower sternomastoid branch of
occipital artery; 18 = facial vein; 19 = accessory nerve;
20 = upper sternomastoid branch of occipital artery;
21 = digastric muscle (posterior belly)

Figure 22.8 Anatomy related to digastric muscle (from RSN, by permission)

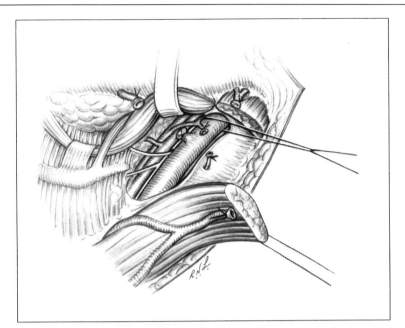

Figure 22.9   Ligation superior end internal jugular vein (from RSN, by permission)

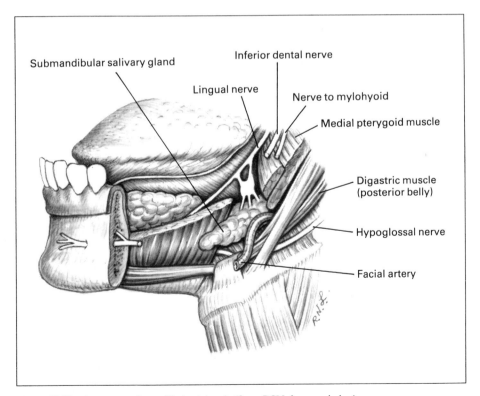

Figure 22.10   Anatomy submandibular triangle (from RSN, by permission)

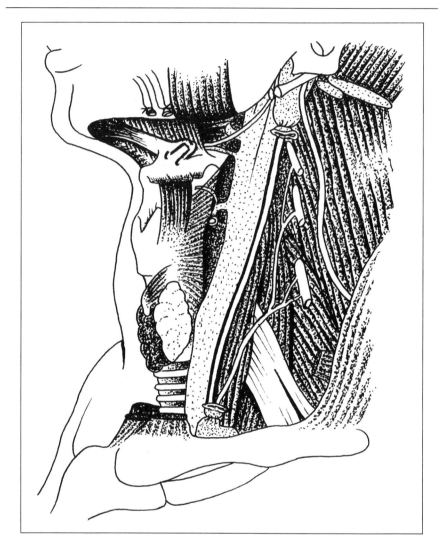

Figure 22.11   Appearance of neck after removal of the neck dissection specimen

Post-operative care

1. The drains should be removed when there is minimal drainage (<10 ml in 24 hours), usually after 24 to 48 hours.
2. Active physiotherapy to the shoulder on the side of the operation should commence when the skin sutures are removed.
3. When the operation is a second side procedure and signs of cerebral oedema develop then intravenous diuretics, such as mannitol, should be used.

Chapter 23

Principles and practice of reconstructive plastic surgery as applied to otolaryngology

SURGERY FOR SKIN LESIONS OF THE NOSE, FACE AND EAR

Introduction

The majority of neoplasms on the face and nose are, by far, basal cell carcinomas. A small percentage are squamous cell carcinoma and there is a small but significantly increasing number of melanoma. On the pinna the numbers of basal cell carcinomas and squamous cell carcinomas are more or less equal.

Indications

Whenever there is a suspicion that a facial or ear lesion may be malignant then excision is generally advised in all but extremely frail individuals.

Specimen

An excisional biopsy should always be performed as opposed to an incisional biopsy. The margin of excision has to be balanced between an adequate tumour-free margin and the cosmesis of the resultant defect. In general, a 5–10 mm of normal skin should be excised. In some circumstances the excision margin has to be tailored to anatomical vital structures, such as the eye, combined with a knowledge of the biological behaviour of the tumour. For example, a basal cell carcinoma close to the eye may require a minimal excision margin, whereas a melanoma which approaches onto the eye will probably require an orbital exenteration.

If there is doubt as to the excision margins of the specimen then biopsies should be taken from the wound bed. The use of frozen section is also advised when there is doubt.

Where adequate pathological facilities are available the technique of Mho's analysis can be employed to achieve adequate excision with minimal cosmetic deformity.

Pre-operative considerations

One should mark the margins of the excision prior to infiltration with local anaesthetic to avoid distortion of resection margins. If a surgeon is doubtful as to the effectiveness of the margin of resection or is uncertain as to the success of a flap repair, a split skin graft or skin to mucosa suture is an acceptable temporary solution which does not usually compromise future flap reconstruction. The planned incision and scar lines should always take account of and lie within lines of relaxation (skin creases) on the face and neck. These creases and folds are highlighted in Figure 23.1 .

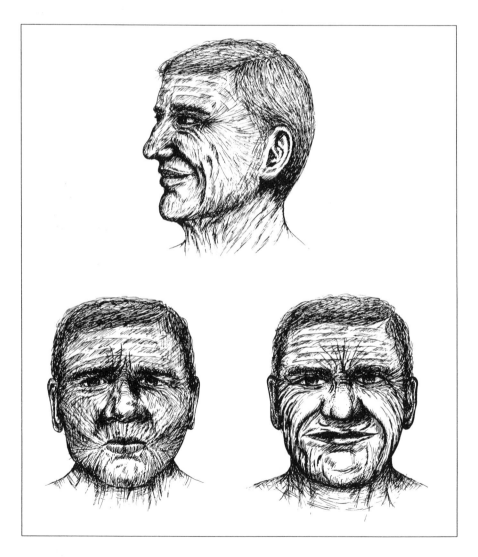

Figure 23.1   Always consider the facial creases as lines of election for skin incisions. After Grabb and Smith

Preparation

For small lesions local anaesthetic (lignocaine 1% with 1:200 000 adrenaline) is appropriate. For larger lesions a general anaesthetic delivered through an oral or nasal endotracheal tube is preferable. If local flaps are planned to be raised during the reconstruction it is preferable to avoid the use of vasoconstrictive agents as they can cause difficulty in the assessment of the flap viability during the reconstruction.

The patient is placed supine on the table with a head ring for support. An aqueous skin preparation which is not injurious to the cornea should be used. If extensive facial surgery is to be performed it is often wiser to perform temporary tarsorrhaphies.

OPERATIONS

Illustrated and described below are various sites of tumour removal and methods of repair.

1. Direct closure

Figure 23.2. Small local lesions can be excised and closed primarily. The line of the scar should be determined by the natural skin crease lines which can be determined by pinching the skin to identify the direction of the natural folds. Fishtail incisions can on occasion simplify closure and diminish dog ears.

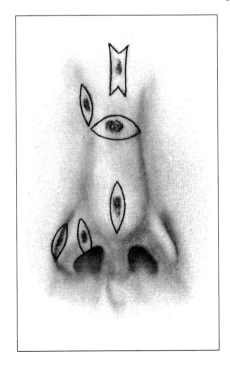

Figure 23.2 Excision of facial skin lesions on the nose (from RSN, by permission)

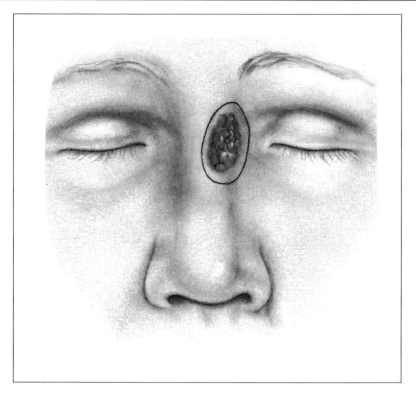

Figure 23.3   Excision planning of a lesion prior to full thickness skin grafting (from RSN, by permission)

2.   Full thickness skin graft

When a defect such as that shown in Figure 23.3 cannot be closed primarily and when there is an adequate vascular base to the defect then a full thickness skin graft can be used. The full thickness skin gives a superior cosmetic result to split skin and is less prone to scar contracture.

A template is made of the size of the defect with the foil of a suture pack. This pattern is now superimposed on the postauricular skin. The addition of a superior and inferior triangle to the pattern facilitates the primary closure of the defect. Figure 23.4 demonstrates the harvesting of a Wolfe or full thickness skin graft. The graft is dissected free and the post auricular wound is closed primarily. Any fat on the deep surface of the graft is trimmed off with blunt curved scissors. The full thickness graft is sutured edge to edge within the defect. Figure 23.5 demonstrates this. Some of the sutures are left long and these are then tied over a pad of proflavine-impregnated cotton wool. This tie over immobilizes the graft. The pad sutures are removed after 1 week.

3.   Composite skin graft

An infiltrative lesion of the columella or alar margin requires full thickness

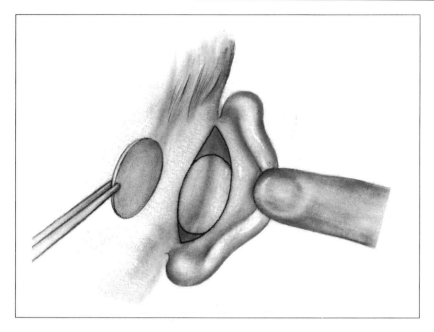

Figure 23.4   Harvest of Wolfe or full thickness graft (from RSN, by permission)

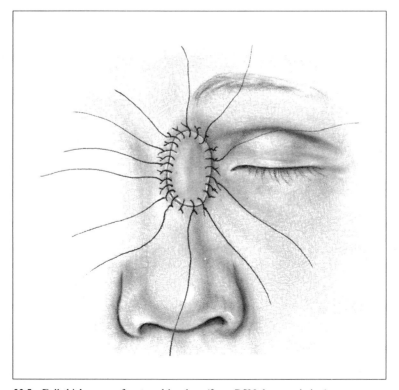

Figure 23.5   Full thickness graft sutured in place (from RSN, by permission)

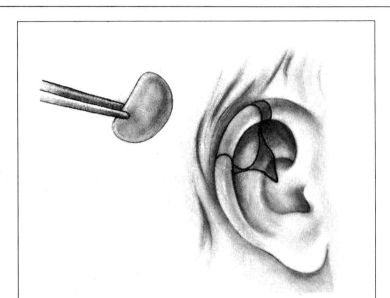

Figure 23.6   Design for harvest of a composite graft (from RSN, by permission)

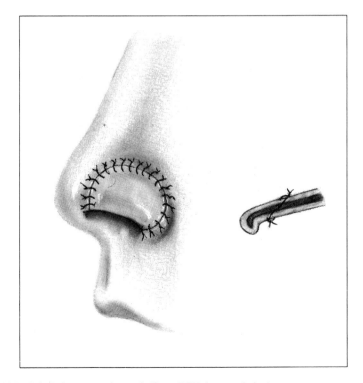

Figure 23.7   Inlay of a composite graft (from RSN, by permission)

excision and if the defect is less than 1 cm in depth then a composite graft of skin and cartilage harvested from the ear is the method of choice.

Following excision of the lesion a three-dimensional mould of the defect is constructed. Dental compound or material used to take impressions for hearing aid moulds can be used. The mould is then transferred to the ear and an appropriate section of the helix chosen.

The graft is marked out and then a wedge is drawn with the apex running into the conchal bowl. The wedge resection from the ear is closed primarily. Figure 23.6 demonstrates these points.

The graft is handled with great care as it receives all its blood supply through the wound margins. Atraumatic careful suturing with interrupted 6-0 proline is required. No dressings are applied. The graft is typically blue for the first 48 hours. Figure 23.7 shows the graft in place.

4. The nasolabial flap

For large alar defects a nasolabial flap is a useful reconstruction. In male patients one should be careful not to transfer the beard onto the nose. Figure 23.8 demonstrates the design of the excision and the flap repair.

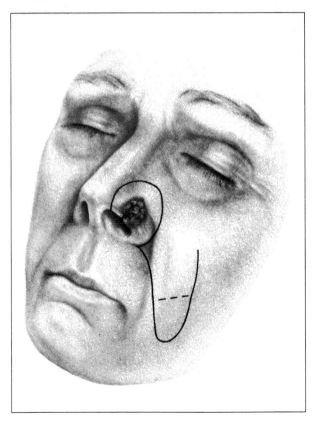

Figure 23.8 Design of a nasolabial flap (from RSN, by permission)

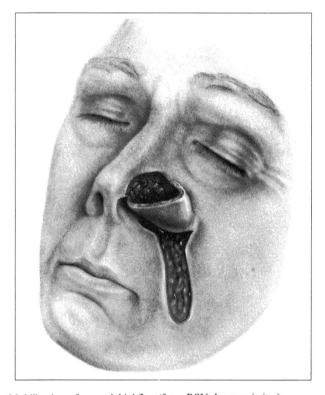

Figure 23.9 Mobilization of a nasolabial flap (from RSN, by permission)

In Figure 23.9 the flap is enfolded to provide both internal and external cover to the nose and adequate support to the nostril.

In Figure 23.10 the donor site has been closed primarily and the flap inset. In some instances revision of the base of the flap to improve the cosmetic appearance is required after 3–6 months.

5.   The glabellar flap

If during the resection of a tumour in the upper third of the nose periosteum is removed then there is an inadequate bed for take of a skin graft and a flap will be required.

Figure 23.11 demonstrates the design of the glabellar flap whereby skin is transferred from the forehead onto the nasal bridge. In Figure 23.12 the flap has been elevated and pivoted on the medial end of the opposite eyebrow and transposed into the defect. The flap is sutured into place and the donor defect closed primarily following minimal undermining.

6.   Wedge excision from the ear

Figure 23.13 demonstrates the planning for a wedge excision to treat a squamous or basal cell carcinoma of the pinna.

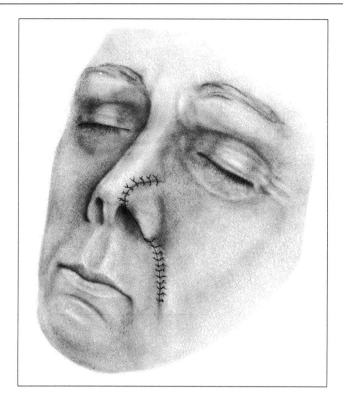

Figure 23.10 Wound closure following nasolabial flap surgery (from RSN, by permission)

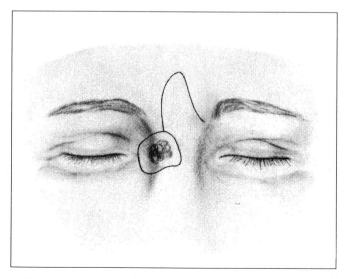

Figure 23.11 Design of a glabellar flap (from RSN, by permission)

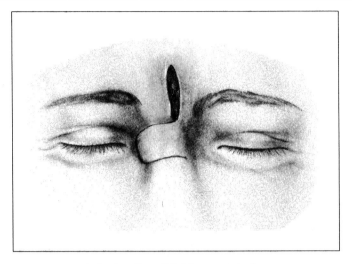

Figure 23.12   Inset of a glabellar flap (from RSN, by permission)

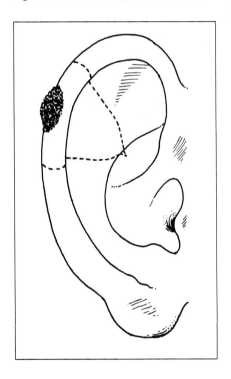

Figure 23.13   Design of wedge resection ear (from RSN, by permission)

Following removal of a lesion with adequate margins closure is performed in layers. The cartilage is first sutured after excision of horizontal wedges sufficient to prevent buckling of the ear. Figure 23.14 demonstrates this point. The skin is sutured with non-absorbable 4-0 or 5-0 prolene.

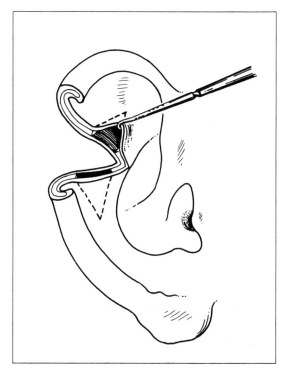

Figure 23.14   Excision of redundant cartilage to facilitate accurate closure (from RSN, by permission)

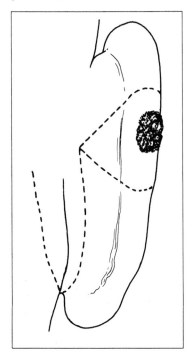

Figure 23.15   Design of a post-auricular transposition flap (from RSN, by permission)

For other lesions on the pinna it may be possible either to excise them and close directly, or if this is not possible to excise and repair with a skin graft and a tie-over dressing as described above in paragraph 2.

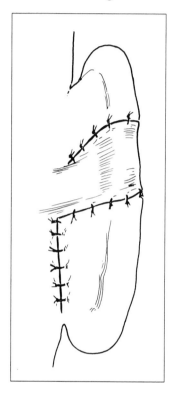

Figure 23.16   Post-auricular closure following transposition (from RSE, by permission)

7.   Transposition flaps on the pinna

For more extensive lesions a transposition flap from the skin taken from the postauricular fold can be effective in repair of the pinna. Figure 23.15 demonstrates the planning of such a procedure. Figure 23.16 and Figure 23.17 demonstrate the result after the flap has been transposed.

GENERAL PRINCIPLES IN THE USE OF FLAPS FOR RECONSTRUCTION

After surgical extirpation of lesions in the head and neck regional flaps are usually preferred to local skin flaps or grafts for reconstruction. These regional flaps have allowed the range of radical surgery to become more extensive. The function of these flaps is:

- To resurface a large skin or mucosal defect.
- To facilitate restoration of function.

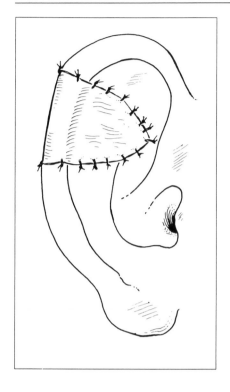

Figure 23.17 The appearance following flap transposition (from RSE, by permission)

- To protect major vital vascular structures such as the carotid arteries.
- To fill out and improve the cosmetic appearance of a defect.

In general one should always begin with the simplest solution and only proceed to use more complex methods when the simple solution is inadequate. There are four principal types of flaps:

1. Random.
2. Axial.
3. Myocutaneous.
4. Free.

1. A random pattern flap has no axial arteriovenous system and derives its blood supply from the communication of vessels in the dermal/subdermal plexus. The viable length of a random flap is related to its width. This differs in various regions of the body. On the face the length-to-width ratio can maximally be about 3:1 or 4:1. On the trunk a ratio of 1:1 is more appropriate.
2. An axial pattern flap has a recognizable arteriovenous circulation that follows the long axis of the flap with branches to the dermal/subdermal plexus. The width-to-length ratio of such a flap does not affect the viability of these flaps. It is the length of the specific axial vessel within the flap that is the most important feature. The deltopectoral flap is a good example of an axial flap.

3.   In a myocutaneous flap there is a rich vascular communication between the muscle and the overlying skin. This allows an entire skin muscle flap to be elevated without regard to the length-and-width ratio as long as the muscle has an adequate circulation. The muscle part of a myocutaneous flap can have either an axial or a random blood supply. In general those muscles with random blood supply do not form good myocutaneous flaps. An example of such a muscle would be the sternocleidomastoid. The best muscles to form myocutaneous flaps are the flat muscles, such as the pectoralis major, trapezius or latissimus dorsi muscles, which have an axial blood supply through a segmental vessel.

4.   The development of microvascular anastomosis has hastened the development of free flaps. A free flap may contain skin, muscle and bone. It can be tailored to the defect in the head and neck which is to be reconstructed. A free flap has an artery and at least one vein which are anastomosed to vessels available in the head and neck. In particular, intra-oral reconstruction has been greatly helped by free flaps. There are a large number of donor sites for free flaps currently described, but the most commonly used in head and neck reconstruction include the radial forearm flap (described later), the groin and iliac crest composite flap and the scapular flap.

Tissue handling of flaps

During the elevation of the reconstructive flaps the tissue which is to be transferred should be handled very carefully. Skin hooks should be used at edges of flaps to minimize damage. Fine sutures should be used to secure vessels on a flap rather than diathermy. Diathermy, even bipolar, can produce extensive thrombosis of associated vessels and place the vascularity of the flap at risk.

It is not possible to discuss all the potential flaps used in head and neck reconstruction. The technique for the use of four common ones will be described. This includes the deltopectoral flap, the pectoralis major flap, the latissimus dorsi flap and a free radial forearm flap.

THE DELTOPECTORAL FLAP

Anatomy

This is a medially based chest flap. Figure 23.18 demonstrates the typical outline of a deltopectoral flap. The blood supply derives from the axial branches of the first four internal mammary perforating vessels. The base of the flap, therefore, straddles the first four intercostal spaces. The upper flap margin is at the level of the clavicle and the lower level runs almost parallel to it as it proceeds from approximately the fifth costochondral junction to the apex of the anterior axillary fold. From there a random extension of the flap can be curved on to the shoulder. When this flap is elevated it is crucial to raise the deep pectoral fascia with the cutaneous flap as the blood supply runs superficial to this fascia.

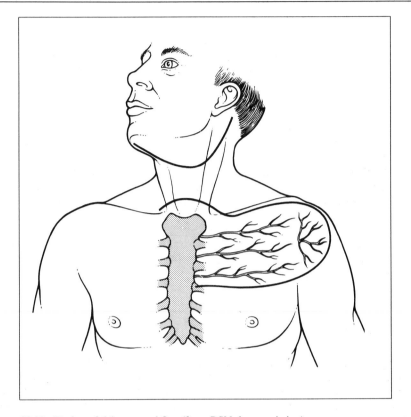

Figure 23.18   Design of deltopectoral flap (from RSN, by permission)

Indications

The deltopectoral flap can be transposed (tubed or untubed, lined or unlined, and delayed or undelayed) to almost any region in the head and neck. It can be used to resurface the chest, neck and face, to reconstruct within the pharynx and oesophageal region and to create a tracheal stoma as well as to provide intra-oral rehabilitation and orbitomaxillary reconstruction.

This flap is often outlined as a surgeon plans a pectoralis major flap under the deltopectoral flap.

Pre-operative considerations

This flap has its greatest range in persons of a stocky build with broad shoulders and a short neck. One should always ensure that the skin of the chest has had neither previous surgery, nor irradiation, prior to planning a delto-pectoral flap.

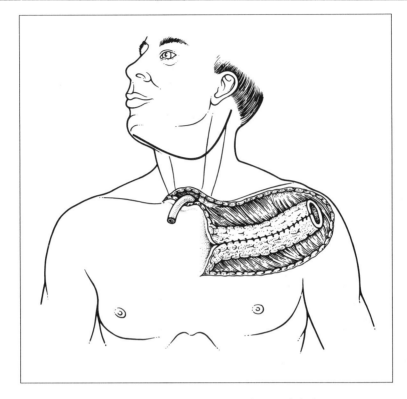

Figure 23.19   Tubing of a deltopectoral flap (from RSN, by permission)

Risks

1. Loss of the flap due to compromise of its vascular supply (discussed above).
2. Separation of the suture repair line as a result of the weight of tissue and dependent position of the flap.
3. Difficulty with healing or scarring on the anterior chest wall.

Method

The flap is first outlined, as demonstrated in Figure 23.18. The flap is elevated from lateral to medial deep to the pectoral fascia to within 1.5 cm of the margin of the sternum. The flap can be tubed with the skin facing outward or with the skin facing inward, as demonstrated in Figure 23.19. The flap is inset into the area for repair with a minimum of tension on the flap.

Post-operative care

Careful observation is required to ensure that no haematoma forms which may compromise the vascularity of the flap. Pressure dressings should never be applied over the pedicle of the flap as this may lead to obstruction of the vascular supply.

After approximately 17–21 days the pedicle of this flap is divided and repositioned into the defect on the chest. The donor site of the flap on the chest is skin grafted either primarily or secondarily, 48 hours after the elevation and rotation of the flap.

PECTORALIS MAJOR FLAP

Anatomy

The pectoralis major muscle is a flat, fan-shaped muscle originating from the medial half of the anterior surface of the clavicle, half the width of the sternum, all the adjacent costal cartilages to the sixth or seventh rib and the aponeurosis of the external/oblique muscle. Pectoralis major inserts by two lamina into the lateral lip of the bicipital groove of the humerus.

The main vascular supply to this axial pattern flap is through the pectoral branch of the thoraco-acromial artery. The lateral thoracic artery and to a minor degree the superior thoracic artery also supply the pectoralis major muscle. This flap can be elevated on its vessel alone, but more typically a narrow strip of muscle is elevated at the same time to protect the arterial pedicle.

Indications

This flap can be used to:

1. Resurface the face and neck.
2. Reconstruct within the oral cavity, oropharynx or hypopharynx.
3. Be used for mandibular reconstruction as an osseomyocutaneous flap. The positioning of a pectoralis major flap in the neck has the advantage of augmenting the contour of the neck and of protecting the carotid artery.

Pre-operative considerations

The design of the flap should preserve the skin of the upper chest, which can be used for primary or secondary resurfacing as a deltopectoral flap. There can be difficulty in contouring this myocutaneous flap in the oral cavity or in the hypopharynx in men who are particularly muscular. Usually in men a skin graft has to be placed in the donor site defect whereas in women the incision can often be closed primarily. Diathermy should be avoided while elevating a myocutaneous flap. Individual vessels which are cut during the elevation of the flap should be clipped and ligated with fine 4-0 chromic catgut.

Risks

1. The skin paddle may be hair-bearing, and in an intra-oral reconstruction this may be troublesome.
2. Fat necrosis is the most serious complication and fortunately is rare. The cause is often not identified, but compression from an overly tight, supraclavicular subcutaneous tunnel as well as vascular pedicle occlusion have been reported.
3. Malposition of the nipple following this surgery may concern patients.

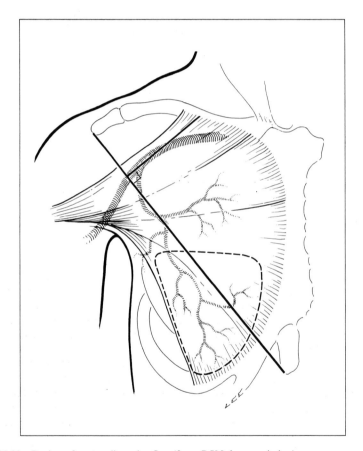

Figure 23.20   Design of pectoralis major flap (from RSN, by permission)

Method

1. Figure 23.20 demonstrates the basic outline for the elevation of a pectoralis major flap. The two key landmarks are the acromial and xiphoid process.

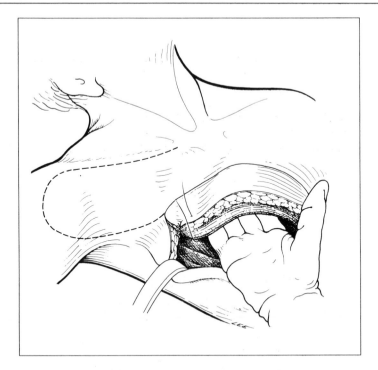

Figure 23.21 Elevation of a pectoralis major flap (from RSN, by permission)

2. A line is drawn between these two points, and then from the mid point of the clavicle a perpendicular line is drawn to meet the original line. The meeting point, as demonstrated in Figure 23.20, marks the line of the acromiothoracic artery. The inferior margin of the pectoralis muscle is identified by palpation and this is used as the lower limit of the area of skin to be marked out.
3. The incision commences at the lower border of the flap to identify correctly the lower margin of the pectoralis major muscle. The skin is stitched to the muscle as the paddle is elevated. A hand can be passed underneath the pectoralis muscle and the vascular supply identified. Figure 23.21 demonstrates a flap being elevated and also the outline of the reserve deltopectoral flap.
4. Figure 23.22 demonstrates the elevation of the deltopectoral flap medially. The protective muscle pedicle overlying the arterial supply to the pectoralis major flap is now dissected free up to the clavipectoral fascia, where the vessel arises from the second part of the axillary artery.
5. As shown in Figure 23.23 a pectoralis muscle flap with the skin stitched to it can now be swung over the clavicle and under the neck skin into wherever the reconstruction is required. It is very important when passing the flap through the neck that the pedicle is not twisted.
6. The donor site on the chest can be either closed primarily, if possible, by undermining surrounding skin widely. Alternatively a skin graft may be

placed over the defect. A suction drain should be inserted at the end of the procedure. The wound should be closed in two layers with a deep layer of absorbable and a cutaneous layer of non-absorbable sutures.

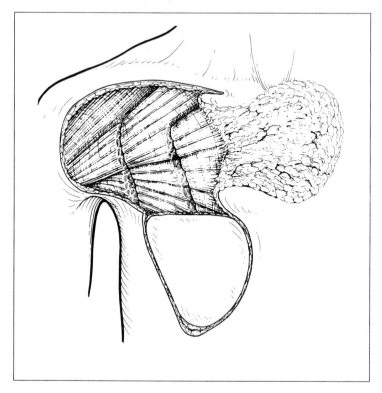

Figure 23.22   Elevation of deltopectoral flap medially with pectoralis major flap designed (from RSN, by permission)

Post-operative care

This will be dependent largely on the procedure for which the pectoralis major flap has been raised. The viability of the flap should always be regularly assessed.

LATISSIMUS DORSI MYOCUTANEOUS FLAP

Anatomy

The latissimus dorsi muscle is flat and arises from the thoracic and lumbar, vertebrae, sacrum and iliac crest and inserts on to the intertubercular groove of the humerus. It receives its axial pattern vascular supply through the thoraco-dorsal artery and vein from the third part of the axillary artery and vein.

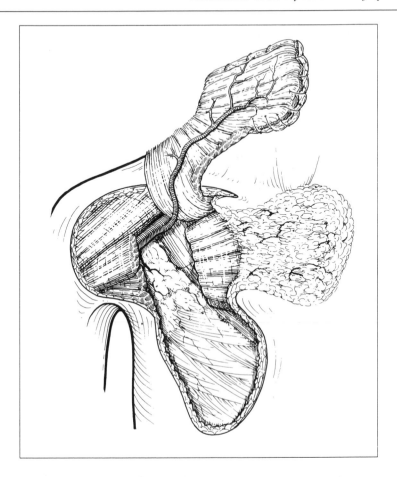

Figure 23.23   Elevation of pectoralis major and deltopectoral flap at the same time (from RSN, by permission)

Indications

This flap is useful for resurfacing the skin of the neck, lower cheek and anterior oral cavity, in addition to augmenting tissue within the cervical region. This flap can be used alone or in combination with other local or regional flaps. Almost invariably this flap provides healthy tissue from a non-irradiated donor site with minimal functional loss and considerable quantity of tissue for transfer. The pedicle often helps to contour the neck after the loss of the sternomastoid muscle from a radical neck dissection.

Pre-operative considerations

There are often considerable difficulties in positioning the patient during the operation. The patient usually starts in the supine position for surgery to the head and neck and is required to be turned over to gain access to the latissimus dorsi flap.

Risks

1. Haematoma at donor site.
2. Necrosis of the flap.
3. When a patient has had a neck dissection and consequently loss of the spinal accessory nerve the use of the latissimus dorsi muscle myocutaneous flap increases shoulder weakness and diminishes shoulder movement. This can worsen shoulder stiffness post-operatively.

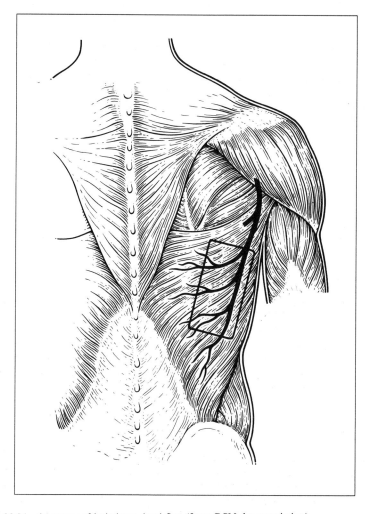

Figure 23.24 Anatomy of latissimus dorsi flap (from RSN, by permission)

Method

1. The plan of the flap is shown in Figure 23.24. To design the flap the distance from the surgical defect to the pectoral/humeral junction is measured along a line curving around the base of the neck. This measured distance is then applied along a line which runs behind the anterior border of the latissimus dorsi down towards its origin from the iliac crest to the area chosen for the flap somewhere between the sixth and tenth rib area. This line will lie superficially over the vascular supply.
2. The incision commences at the mid-portion of the vascular pedicle and a plane of dissection is created between serratus anterior and the latissimus dorsi muscle.
3. The flap is elevated in a distal to proximal direction with preservation of the vascular pedicle following the division of the muscle superiorly. A tunnel is created deep to the anterior axillary wall through the clavipectoral fascia, then superficial to the clavicle and thus the flap is led into the neck wound. The flap should be inset into the defect without tension or torsion.
4. The donor site can usually be closed primarily following undermining of the local tissues. A suction drain should be inserted into the donor site and the repair of the donor defect should be in two layers with an absorbable suture deep, and a non-absorbable suture to the skin.

Post-operative care

1. The viability of the flap should always be monitored.
2. The drains should be removed from the donor site when there is a

RADIAL FOREARM FREE FLAP

Anatomy

The radial forearm flap is a fasciocutaneous flap that includes volar forearm skin, the underlying fascia and the intermuscular fascia which contains the radial artery and its cutaneous branches. The venous drainage of this flap can be either via the superficial veins, such as the cephalic vein, or with the communicating veins which run with the radial artery. The radial artery arises from the brachial artery within the antecubital fossa and lengths of the radial artery up to 20 cm can be harvested. The radial forearm bone can sometimes be contained within a radial forearm flap.

Indications

This flap is particularly useful in the oral cavity as the skin is thin, pliable and hairless. It is especially useful for small defects in the anterior oral cavity in which the import of tissue is required to maintain tongue mobility and oral function but where bulk may be a disadvantage. The flap contours well within the oral cavity and naturally, unlike pedicled flaps, it is unaffected by gravity.

In the illustrations shown, however, the flap has been tubed to be used for pharyngeal reconstruction.

Pre-operative considerations

Prior to raising the flap the arterial supply to the hand must be assessed, either clinically using the Allen test (compression of the radial artery and ulnar artery at the wrist) or by the use of a doppler ultrasound examination. This should determine that the ulnar arterial supply to the whole hand is adequate.

Risks

1. Failure of the flap.
2. Delayed healing as a result of skin graft failure at the donor site. The incidence of this problem can be reduced by avoiding skin from the distal forearm and careful preservation of the paratenon, which reduces the likelihood of this problem occurring.
3. Donor site scarring can be a problem, particularly in women patients.
4. Swelling of the hand or the wrist may occur and it is usual for up to 3 weeks. On occasion the swelling may continue for up to 3 months.
5. Cold-induced symptoms and reduced or abnormal sensation in all or part of the radial nerve distribution may occur post-operatively.
6. If bone has been included in the flap the donor site must be immobilized for at least 4 to 6 weeks since there is a risk of a pathological fracture.

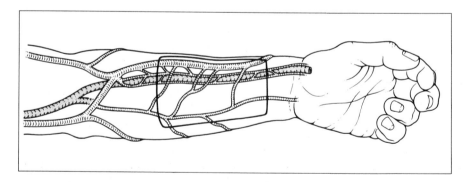

Figure 23.25 Anatomy of radial forearm flap (from RSN, by permission)

Method

1. Figure 23.25 shows the outline of the flap.
2. The incisions are carried down on to the muscular fascia and the flaps elevated subfascially from both the medial and lateral sides towards the fascial mesentery which conducts the arteries. The distal vessels are divided and ligated. Proximally the vessels are exposed almost up to the antecubital

fossa in order to provide a length of pedicle for the microvascular anastomosis.

3. Once the flap is elevated an assessment of the flap circulation is made and it is then wrapped in a warm saline gauze to await detachment. When the recipient site is prepared the radial vessels and cephalic vein are transected and the flap transferred. The proximal vessels which are to be anastomosed should not have clamps placed upon them. The flap should be flushed through with a heparin/saline solution, which is best done with a syringe and blunt needle.

4. The skin paddle may be used as a patch for oropharyngeal repair or tubed, as demonstrated in Figure 23.26, prior to transfer for pharyngeal repair.

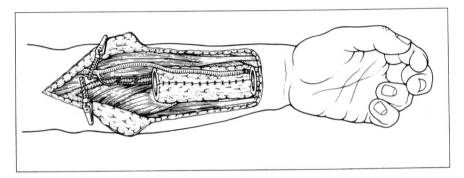

Figure 23.26 Radial forearm flap tubed (from RSN, by permission)

5. The donor site can often be closed partly primarily, but usually a skin graft is required with a tie-over dressing supporting the graft.

6. The flap is sutured in place before the microvascular anastomosis is completed. It is important that a pharyngeal reconstruction is not under excessive tension.

7. Figure 23.27 demonstrates the free flap in position with the anastomoses. The most effective vascular anastomosis is end to side and if possible the external carotid artery is chosen. In the presence of excessive atheroma the facial or superior thyroid arteries may be chosen. The microvascular anastomosis should not be under tension. Ideally the internal jugular vein is appropriate for the venous anastomosis, but this has often been excised during radical neck dissection. In this situation the external or anterior jugular vein is appropriate.

The anastomoses are performed using the operating microscope and atraumatic 8-0 or 9-0 nylon or prolene.

Post-operative care

It is important to assess the viability of the free flap at regular intervals following the surgery. Failure in the viability of the flap requires a return to the operating room.

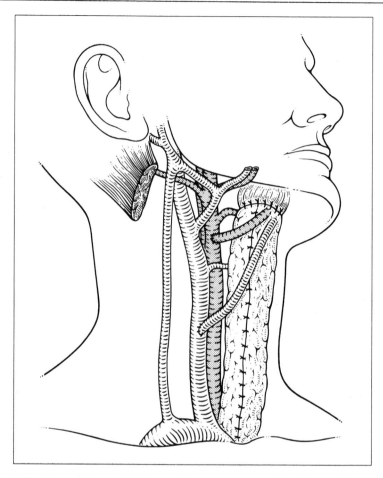

Figure 23.27   The use of a radial forearm flap to reconstruct the pharynx (from RSN, by permission)

Appendix: list of suppliers

The following list of companies supplied materials to the authors' surgical department:

Aesculop 3 March Place Gatehouse Way Aylesbury Bucks HP19 3DB UK	Instruments
Cochlear Pty Ltd 14 Mars Road Lane Cove NSW 2066 Australia	Cochlear implants
Coherent Medical Division 3270 West Bayshore Road PO Box 10321 Palo Alto California 94303 USA	CO_2 laser
Dow Corning Kings Court 185 Kings Road Reading Berks RG1 4EX UK	Thin silastic sheeting
Ethicon PO Box 408 Edinburgh EH11 4HE UK	Sutures
Exmoor Plastics Ltd Lisieux Way Taunton Somerset TA1 2LB UK	Splints Ventilation tubes

Gebrueder Martin   UK Distributor: Albert Waeschle   Instruments
72 Tuttlingen/Postfach 60   PO Box 19
Germany   123–125 Old
                                          Christchurch Road
                                          Bournemouth
                                          BH1 1EX

John Weiss and Son Ltd 89 Alston Drive Bradwell Abbey Milton Keynes Bucks MK13 9HF UK			Instruments
Karl Storz GMBH and Co Mittelstrasse 8 Postfach 230 D-7200 Tuttlingon Germany	UK Distributor:	Rimmer Brothers Aylesbury House Clerkenwell Green London EC1R 0DD	Endoscopy equipment
Ketac-cem ESPE Fabrik Pharmazeutischer Präparate GMBH and Co KG D-8031 Seefeld/Oberbay Germany			Cement
Microtek Medical Inc. Post Office Box 2487 Columbus Mississippi USA	UK Distributor	Hartwell Medical Ltd. Unit 27 Croft Road Newcastle-under- Lyme ST5 0TW	Drapes Middle ear implants
Regent LRC Products Ltd London E4 8QA UK			Surgical gloves
Richard Wolf UK Ltd PO Box 47 Mitcham Surrey CR4 4TT UK			Endoscopy equipment
Shiley Ltd Shiley House 42 Thames Street Windsor Berks SL4 1PR UK			Tracheostomy tubes
Smith and Nephew Richards 6 The Technopark Newmarket Road Cambridge CB5 8PB UK		Richards Medical Co. 1450 Brooks Road Memphis TN38116 USA	Instruments Middle ear implants Cochlear implants

Xomed-Treace	Xomed-Treace	Middle ear
Zimmer	6743 Southpoint	implants
Surgitek	Drive North	Instruments
Hall	Jacksonville	Facial nerve
Dunbeath Road	Florida 32216	stimulator
Elgin Industrial Estate	USA	
Swindon		
SN2 6EA		
UK		
Zeiss		Operating
Carl Zeiss		microscope
D-7082 Oberkochen		
Germany		

Index